CLINICAL
SKILLBUILDERS™

S0-BBF-105

I.V. Therapy

C L I N I C A L
SKILLBUILDERS™

I.V. Therapy

Springhouse Corporation
Springhouse, Pennsylvania

STAFF

Executive Director, Editorial
Stanley Loeb

Editorial Director
Matthew Cahill

Clinical Director
Barbara F. McVan, RN

Art Director
John Hubbard

Senior Editor
William J. Kelly

Clinical Editors
Maryann Foley, RN, BSN; Judith A. Schilling McCann, RN, BSN

Editors
Barbara Delp, Margaret Eckman, Doris Falk, Karla Harby, Elizabeth Mauro

Copy Editors
Jane V. Cray (supervisor), Mary Durkin, Nancy Papsin, Doris Weinstock

Designers
Stephanie Peters (associate art director),

Matie Patterson (senior designer), Julie Carlton Barlow, Linda Franklin

Illustrators
Jean Gardner, Frank Grobelny, Robert Jackson, John Murphy, Robert Neumann, Judy Newhouse, Wendy Wray

Art Production
Robert Perry (manager), Anna Brindisi, Donald Knauss, Thomas Robbins, Robert Wieder

Typography
David Kosten (director), Diane Paluba (manager), Elizabeth Bergman, Joyce Rossi Biletz, Phyllis Marron, Robin Rantz, Valerie Rosenberger

Manufacturing
Deborah Meiris (manager), T.A. Landis, Jennifer Suter

Production Coordination
Aline S. Miller (manager), Maura Murphy

Editorial Assistants
Maree DeRosa, Beverly Lane, Mary Madden

©1990 by Springhouse Corporation, 1111 Bethlehem Pike, P.O. Box 908, Springhouse, Pa. 19477-0908. All rights reserved. Reproduction in whole or part by any means whatsoever without written permission of the publisher is prohibited by law. Authorization to photocopy any items for internal or personal use, or the internal or personal use of specific clients, is granted by Springhouse Corporation for users registered with the Copyright Clearance Center (CCC) Transactional Reporting Service, provided that the base fee of $00.00 per copy plus $.75 per page is paid directly to CCC, 27 Congress St., Salem, Mass. 01970. For those organizations that have been granted a license by CCC, a separate system of payment has been arranged. The fee code for users of the Transactional Reporting Service is 087434350X/90 $00.00 + $.75.
Printed in the United States of America.
CS3-050893

Library of Congress
Cataloging-in-Publication Data
I.V therapy
         p. cm. – (Clinical Skillbuilders™)
    Includes bibliographical references and index.
    1. Intravenous therapy – Handbooks, manuals, etc.   2. Nursing-Handbooks, manuals, etc.   I. Springhouse Corporation. II. Series.
    [DNLM: 1. Infusions, Intravenous – handbooks.   2. Infusions, Intravenous – nurses' instruction.   WB 39 I93
RM170.I2   1991
615.8'55 – dc20
DNLM/DLC   90-10409
ISBN 0-87434-350-X

CONTENTS

ADVISORY BOARD AND CONTRIBUTORS

At the time of publication, the advisors held the following positions.

Sandra G. Crandall, RN,C, MSN, CRNP
Director
Center for Nursing Excellence
Newtown, Pa.

Terry Matthew Foster, RN, BSN, CEN, CCRN
Clinical Director, Nursing Administration
Mercy Hospital-Anderson
Cincinnati
Staff Nurse, Emergency Department
Saint Elizabeth Medical Center
Covington, Ky.

Sandra K. Goodnough-Hanneman, RN, PhD
Critical Care Consultant, Nursing
Houston

Doris A. Millam, RN, MS, CRNI
I.V. Therapy Clinician
Holy Family Hospital
Des Plaines, Ill.

Deborah Panozzo Nelson, RN, MS, CCRN
Cardiovascular Clinical Specialist
Visiting Assistant Professor
EMS Nursing Education
Purdue University, Calumet Campus
Hammond, Ind.

Marilyn Sawyer Sommers, RN, PhD, CCRN
Assistant Professor
College of Nursing and Health
University of Cincinnati

At the time of publication, the contributors held the following positions.

Joan M. Baumann, RN, MA, CCRN
Critical Care Clinical Instructor
Holy Cross Hospital
Silver Spring, Md.

Ann M. Corrigan, RN, BSN, MS, CRNI
Nurse Manager
Manchester Memorial Hospital
Manchester, Conn.

Faye Cosentino, RN, BS, CRNI
Director, I.V. Therapy
Lawrence Hospital
Bronxville, N.Y.

Maryann Foley, RN, BSN
Independent Nurse Consultant
Flourtown, Pa.

Mary Ellen Haisfield, RN, MS
Senior Clinical Nurse
The Johns Hopkins Hospital
Baltimore

Judith A. Schilling McCann, RN, BSN
Clinical Editor
Springhouse Corporation
Springhouse, Pa.

Doris A. Millam, RN, MS, CRNI
I.V. Therapy Clinician
Holy Family Hospital
Des Plaines, Ill.

Nancy L. Peck, RN, MSN, CRNI
Nursing Care Coordinator
Thomas Jefferson University Hospital
Philadelphia

Brenda K. Shelton, RN, MS, CCRN, OCN
Critical Care Instructor
The Johns Hopkins Oncology Center
Baltimore

Sharon M. Weinstein, RN, MS, CRNI
Divisional Director of Infusion Therapy
Kimberly Quality Care, Central Division
Winthrop Harbor, Ill.

For most nurses, I.V. therapy used to mean little more than hanging bags of I.V. solutions to maintain fluid balance. But times have changed.

Today, you may be called upon to infuse medications, transfuse blood, or provide parenteral nutrition. What's more, you may be asked to insert a peripheral I.V. line, or to assist with the insertion of a central line or an implanted vascular access device.

Other changes have taken place too. Because of technological advances, patients now commonly receive I.V. therapy in long-term care facilities and at home. So no matter where you work, you need certain I.V. therapy skills. For instance, you need to know how to start an infusion, how to assess a patient during therapy, and how to discontinue the infusion. You also need a broad understanding of I.V. therapy—the different administration methods and their indications, advantages, and disadvantages.

Altogether, that's a lot to learn. But *I.V. Therapy* makes learning easy. This latest volume in the Clinical Skillbuilders™ series tells you all you need to know to manage I.V. therapy with skill and confidence.

A handy pocket-manual, *I.V. Therapy* is designed to be used on the job. The clear writing and logical organization make it easy to consult when time is at a premium. And the book is packed with practical explanations covering all aspects of I.V. therapy.

This new volume consists of seven chapters, with the first offering an overview of the topic and a thorough explanation of fluid and electrolyte balance. The other six chapters focus on administering I.V. therapy to the hospitalized adult patient, though they also address the special needs of pediatric, elderly, and home care patients.

Chapters 2, 3, and 4 examine the different ways to deliver I.V. therapy. Chapter 2 covers peripheral I.V. therapy; Chapter 3, central venous therapy; and Chapter 4, vascular devices implanted under the skin. Each chapter takes you through patient preparation, equipment selection, and the steps for initiating, maintaining, and discontinuing therapy.

The last three chapters explain specific I.V. therapies. Chapter 5 covers administering I.V. medications. Here, you'll review how to use the three main delivery methods: direct injection, intermittent infusion, and continuous infusion. Chapter 6 spells out how to transfuse blood and blood components safely. You'll learn the benefit of each component and gain a better understanding of the importance of routine blood typing. In Chapter 7, you'll find a thorough explanation of parenteral nutrition, including practical advice on how to assess your patient's nutritional status. These three chapters show you step-by-step how to prepare and administer the different solutions. You'll also learn which adverse reactions to watch for and how to handle them when they occur.

Throughout the book, you'll find special graphic symbols, or logos, that indicate certain key recurring topics. For instance, each time you see the *Troubleshooting* logo, you'll find information on detecting and correcting problems with I.V. equipment. The *Complications* logo alerts you to essential information on recognizing, preventing, and treating adverse reactions to therapy.

Short lists of key points to remember about a particular subject carry the *Checklist* logo. In the second chapter, for example, this logo accompanies a list of tips on how to prevent problems with infusion pumps. You'll also find an *Equipment* logo that signals illustrations and explanations of various pieces of I.V. equipment. Plus, the book contains other illustrations, charts, and supplementary text pieces that will enhance your understanding of I.V. therapy.

After you've read the book, you can test your knowledge. Following Chapter 7, you'll find a multiple-choice self-test that focuses on important topics contained in *I.V. Therapy*. An answer key follows the test.

Four helpful appendices follow the self-test. The first provides a listing of common abbreviations you'll encounter when administering I.V. therapy. The second appendix, a chart, lets you check drug compatibility at a glance. The third appendix explains how to measure central venous pressure. And the last appendix is a nomogram for estimating body surface area in children—a key consideration when calculating pediatric drug dosages.

With all this useful information packed into a portable manual, *I.V. Therapy* is an essential tool for all nurses—no matter how experienced. Whether you're learning about I.V. therapy for the first time or you're reviewing key concepts and sharpening your skills, this volume will prove invaluable. I recommend that you read it at home, then take it to work and put it to use.

Jeanette Barnes RN, MS, CRNI, CS
Corporate Director, Infusion and
High-Tech Services
Kimberly Quality Care
Atlanta

1
INTRODUCTION

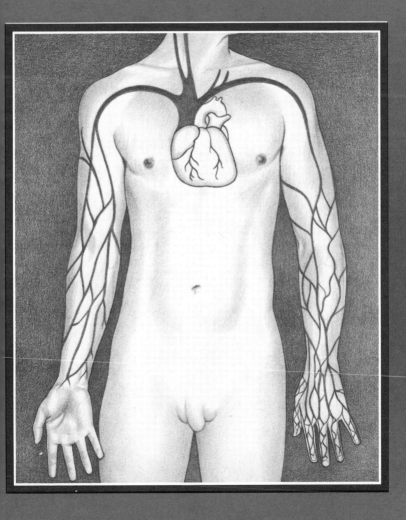

Today, more than 80% of all hospitalized patients receive some form of I.V. therapy. And I.V therapy takes many forms, with more than 200 commercially prepared I.V. fluids now available.

Of course, I.V. nurses play a major role in administering this therapy. But medical-surgical and other nurses are responsible for its hour-to-hour maintenance and, in some hospitals, for initiating certain kinds of I.V. therapy. So you must know how to administer I.V. therapy safely and correctly.

In this chapter, you'll become familiar with I.V. administration methods and primary uses of I.V. therapy. You'll also review the basics of fluid and electrolyte balance. Then you'll cover some fundamentals of administration—how to control infection and how to maintain I.V. flow rates. Finally, you'll read about special considerations in I.V. therapy: legal implications, documentation, patient teaching, and home care.

Basics of I.V. therapy

The principal uses of I.V. therapy include restoring and maintaining fluid and electrolyte balance, administering medications, transfusing blood, and delivering parenteral nutrition solutions.

Depending on the purpose and the specific situation, you may administer I.V. therapy either continuously or intermittently. Continuous I.V. therapy allows you to give a carefully regulated amount of fluid over a prolonged period. For this type of therapy, you may use a peripheral I.V. line or a central venous (CV) line.

In intermittent I.V. therapy, a solution (often a medication) is given for shorter periods at varying intervals. For instance, a small volume—say, 25 to 250 ml—may be given over several minutes or a few hours. With this type of therapy, you may use a winged infusion set, an intermittent injection cap (heparin lock), existing peripheral or CV lines established for continuous infusion, or an implanted venous access device.

Delivery methods
The choice of delivery method depends not only on the purpose and duration of therapy but also on the patient's condition, age, and health history and on the condition of his veins. At times, a patient may receive I.V. therapy by more than one delivery method. For each method, you'll need certain clinical skills to start, maintain, and discontinue therapy.

Peripheral I.V. therapy. With this method, you'll administer I.V. solutions through a vein in the arm or hand or, occasionally, the leg or foot. The site must be easy to sterilize, and the patient must cooperate so you can insert and maintain the I.V. line. (See *Peripheral and central veins used in I.V. therapy.*)

Typically, this method of delivery will be used for short-term (less than 4 weeks) or intermittent therapy. You'll probably administer isotonic fluids—including most medications and parenteral nutrition solutions with a concentration of 12.5% or less—by peripheral I.V. therapy.

CV therapy. With this method, you'll administer I.V. solutions through a central vein, such as the right or left subclavian or the inter-

Peripheral and central veins used in I.V. therapy

This illustration shows the veins commonly used for peripheral I.V. and central venous therapy.

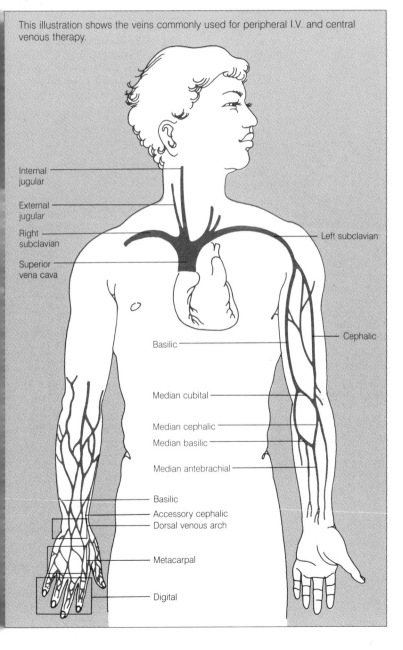

nal or external jugular. Delivery through central veins increases the risk of infection for two reasons. A CV catheter usually remains in place for a long time, and a patient requiring such therapy will probably be immunocompromised.

You'll use this method when a patient needs a large volume of fluid or when the fluid is a hypertonic solution, a caustic drug, or a high-calorie parenteral nutrition solution with a concentration greater than 12.5%. This method may also be used in an emergency when a patient has inaccessible peripheral veins or when a patient needs long-term therapy at home.

Implanted vascular access device. In this variation of CV infusion, the infused solution enters a central vein through an access device that's surgically implanted in a subcutaneous pocket. The device consists of a port with a self-sealing system connected to an outlet catheter. To administer therapy, you need a special needle that passes through the skin and into the port.

You'll see this method of delivery ordered when a patient needs long-term (months to years) I.V. therapy. When used for purposes other than I.V. therapy, this device can also be implanted epidurally, intra-arterially, and intraperitoneally.

Uses of I.V. therapy

Besides maintaining and restoring fluid and electrolyte balance, the most common uses of I.V. therapy include administering drugs, transfusing blood, and delivering parenteral nutrition.

Drug administration. The I.V. route provides a rapid, effective way of administering drugs. Commonly infused drugs include antibiotics, thrombolytics, histamine-receptor antagonists, and antineoplastic, cardiovascular, and anticonvulsant drugs. Usually, you'll give an I.V. drug over a short period—in some cases, by a direct injection (also called I.V. push). You may dilute the drug in 0.9% sodium chloride (normal saline solution) or dextrose 5% in water.

Transfusion. Your nursing responsibilities include administering blood and blood components as well as monitoring patients receiving transfusion therapy. Transfusion aims to maintain adequate blood volume, prevent cardiogenic shock, increase the blood's oxygen-carrying capacity, and maintain hemostasis.

Parenteral nutrition. Parenteral nutrition means giving nutrients by the I.V. route. As mentioned, you'll give a low-concentration parenteral nutrition solution through a peripheral vein but a more highly concentrated one through a central vein. The concentration depends on the nutrients in the particular solution.

Solutions developed for total parenteral nutrition (TPN) provide all of a patient's energy and nutrient requirements: proteins, carbohydrates, fats, electrolytes, vitamins, trace elements, and water. A patient's peripheral veins can't tolerate the high concentrations of amino acids and glucose in these solutions, so you have to use a central vein. A patient can receive TPN through a central vein indefinitely.

Solutions delivered by peripheral veins provide a more limited form of nutritional therapy. They contain fewer nonprotein calories and lower amino acid concentrations, and may include fat. You can use peripheral vein nutrition only for periods of less than 3 weeks to maintain the

CHECKLIST

Identifying fluid imbalances

By carefully assessing a patient receiving I.V. therapy, you can identify fluid imbalances early—before serious complications develop.

FLUID DEFICIT

These assessment findings indicate a fluid deficit:
• weight loss
• lowered body temperature (if infection isn't present)
• increased or decreased pulse rate
• diminished blood pressure, often with postural hypotension
• decreased central venous pressure
• sunken eyes, dry conjunctiva, decreased tearing
• poor skin turgor (not a reliable sign in elderly patients)
• lack of moisture in groin and axillae
• decreased salivation
• dry, cracked lips
• furrows in tongue
• difficulty forming words (patient needs to moisten mouth first)
• cold limbs (with severe fluid volume deficit)
• indifferent attitude
• diminished urine output.
    You may also note these laboratory test results:
• increased hematocrit
• elevated serum electrolyte and blood urea nitrogen (BUN) levels
• increased serum osmolarity.

FLUID EXCESS

These assessment findings indicate a fluid excess:
• weight gain
• elevated blood pressure
• bounding pulse that's not easily obliterated
• jugular vein distention
• increased respiratory rate
• dyspnea
• moist crackles or rhonchi on auscultation
• edema of dependent body parts; sacral edema in patients on bed rest
• good skin turgor
• puffy eyelids
• fuller-than-normal cheeks
• periorbital edema
• hoarseness
• slow emptying of hand veins when arm is raised.
    You may also note these laboratory test results:
• lowered hematocrit
• decreased serum electrolyte levels
• decreased BUN levels
• reduced serum osmolarity.

nutritional status of a patient who doesn't have to gain weight.

    If you're responsible for a patient who's receiving parenteral nutrition, you'll need to know how to recognize changes in fluid and electrolyte status and in glucose, amino acid, mineral, and vitamin levels. You'll also need to judge your patient's response to the nutrient solution and detect early signs of complications.

Fluid and electrolyte balance

Any solution given I.V. can alter a patient's fluid and electrolyte balance. (See *Identifying fluid imbalances*.) So you need to anticipate the fluid and electrolyte changes your patient will experience during therapy and recognize inappropriate orders for I.V. solutions.

Fundamentals of fluid and electrolyte balance

Fluid balance and electrolyte balance are so interdependent that any change in one alters the other. Both fluid and electrolytes continuously move within the body. So fluid and electrolyte balance involves the movement as well as the composition of body fluids. To fully understand this important concept, first review some fundamentals.

Water, the essential component of body fluid, has many functions. It helps regulate body temperature, transports nutrients and gases, carries body wastes to excretion sites, and helps maintain cell shape. Electrolytes, which are also essential, are chemical compounds that dissociate in solution into charged particles (or ions). The electrical charge the ions carry conducts the current necessary for normal cell function (see *Understanding the major electrolytes*).

Body fluid compartments

Within the body, fluid exists in two major compartments, separated by capillary walls and cell membranes. Two-thirds of the fluid exists inside the cells and is called *intracellular fluid* (ICF). The other third exists outside the cells and is known as *extracellular fluid* (ECF). For fluid balance, the distribution between these two compartments must remain relatively constant.

In an adult, the ICF totals 28 liters, accounting for about 40% of total body weight. The ECF totals 14 liters, accounting for about 20%. The ECF consists of *interstitial*

fluid (ISF), which bathes the cells, and *plasma,* the liquid component of blood. In an adult, ISF represents about 75% of ECF; plasma, about 25% (see *Understanding body fluid distribution,* page 9).

A small amount of body fluid— such as cerebrospinal fluid, lymph, and fluids within such spaces as the pleural and abdominal cavities—is considered transcellular.

Fluid distribution varies with age. Infants, for instance, have a greater percentage of body fluid stored in the interstitial space than do adults. This percentage declines until puberty, when the distribution reaches adult levels. As a person ages, his total body fluid, ICF, and ISF all decrease, but the percentage of body weight represented by plasma remains stable.

Electrolyte distribution. The ICF and ECF contain different electrolytes because the cell membranes separating these two compartments have selective permeability. That is, the membranes allow only certain ions to move in and out. The major intracellular electrolytes are potassium and phosphorus; the major extracellular electrolytes, sodium and chloride.

The two ECF components, ISF and plasma, have identical electrolyte compositions. That's because pores in the capillary walls separating them allow free passage of electrolytes. Keep in mind, however, an important difference between ISF and plasma: protein content. Plasma has a fairly high concentration of proteins. But because protein molecules are too large to pass through capillary walls, ISF contains none.

Concentration and osmolarity. Concentration refers to the number of dissolved particles (or solutes) in

Understanding the major electrolytes

Electrolytes dissociate in solution into electrically charged particles called ions that have either a negative charge (anions) or a positive charge (cations). Within each body compartment, the number of cations must equal the number of anions to achieve a chemical balance. A loss or gain of electrolytes and an increase or decrease in body fluid can affect this delicate chemical balance.

Six major electrolytes play important roles in maintaining chemical balance. Electrolyte concentrations are expressed in milliequivalents (mEq) and millimoles (mmol).

ELECTROLYTE	PRINCIPAL FUNCTIONS	SIGNS AND SYMPTOMS OF IMBALANCE
Sodium (Na^+) • Major cation in extra-cellular fluid (ECF) • Normal serum level: 135 to 147 mEq/liter (135 to 147 mmol/L)	• Maintains appropriate ECF osmolarity • Influences water distribution (with chloride) • Affects concentration, excretion, and absorption of potassium and chloride • Helps regulate acid-base balance • Aids nerve- and muscle-fiber impulse transmission	*Hyponatremia:* muscle weakness, decreased skin turgor, headache, tremor, seizures *Hypernatremia:* thirst, fever, flushed skin, oliguria, and dry, sticky membranes
Potassium (K^+) • Major cation in intra-cellular fluid (ICF) • Normal serum level: 3.5 to 5.0 mEq/liter (3.5 to 5.0 mmol/L)	• Maintains cell electroneutrality • Maintains cell osmolarity • Assists in conduction of nerve impulses • Directly affects cardiac muscle contraction • Plays major role in acid-base balance	*Hypokalemia:* decreased GI, skeletal muscle, and cardiac muscle function; decreased reflexes; rapid, weak, irregular pulse; muscle weakness or irritability; decreased blood pressure; nausea and vomiting; paralytic ileus *Hyperkalemia:* muscle weakness, nausea, diarrhea, oliguria
Calcium (Ca^{++}) • Major cation in teeth and bones • Normal serum level: 4 to 5.5 mEq/liter (2 to 2.75 mmol/L)	• Enhances bone strength and durability (along with phosphorus) • Helps maintain cell-membrane structure, function, and permeability • Affects activation, excitation, and contraction of cardiac and skeletal muscles • Participates in neurotransmitter release at synapses • Helps activate specific steps in blood coagulation • Activates serum complement in immune system function	*Hypocalcemia:* muscle tremor, muscle cramps, tetany, tonic-clonic seizures, paresthesia, bleeding, arrhythmias, hypotension *Hypercalcemia:* lethargy, headache, muscle flaccidity, nausea, vomiting, anorexia, constipation, polydipsia, hypertension, polyuria

(continued)

Understanding the major electrolytes *(continued)*

ELECTROLYTE	PRINCIPAL FUNCTIONS	SIGNS AND SYMPTOMS OF IMBALANCE
Chloride (Cl^-) • Major anion in ECF • Normal serum level: 95 to 105 mEq/liter (95 to 105 mmol/L)	• Maintains serum osmolarity (along with Na^+) • Combines with major cations to create important compounds, such as sodium chloride (NaCl), hydrogen chloride (HCl), potassium chloride (KCl), and calcium chloride ($CaCl_2$)	*Hypochloremia:* increased muscle excitability, tetany, decreased respirations *Hyperchloremia:* stupor, rapid deep breathing, muscle weakness
Phosphorus (P^{--}) • Major anion in ICF • Normal serum level (phosphate level): 2.5 to 5.0 mEq/dl (0.80 to 1.60 mmol/L)	• Helps maintain bones and teeth • Helps maintain cell integrity • Plays major role in acid-base balance (as a urinary buffer) • Promotes energy transfer to cells • Plays essential role in muscle, red blood cell, and neurologic functions	*Hypophosphatemia:* paresthesia (circumoral and peripheral), lethargy, speech defects (such as stuttering or stammering) *Hyperphosphatemia:* renal failure, vague neuroexcitability to tetany and convulsions, arrhythmias and muscle twitching with sudden rise in phosphate levels
Magnesium (Mg^{++}) • Major cation in ICF (closely related to Ca^{++} and P^{--}) • Normal serum level: 1.3 to 2.1 mEq/liter (0.65 to 1.05 mmol/L) with 33% bound to protein and remainder as free cations	• Activates intracellular enzymes; active in carbohydrate and protein metabolism • Acts on myoneural junction, affecting neuromuscular irritability and contractility of cardiac and skeletal muscles • Affects peripheral vasodilation • Facilitates Na^+ and K^+ movement across all membranes • Influences Ca^{++} levels	*Hypomagnesemia:* dizziness, confusion, convulsions, tremor, leg and foot cramps, hyperirritability, arrhythmias, vasomotor changes, anorexia, nausea *Hypermagnesemia:* drowsiness, lethargy, coma, arrhythmias, hypotension, vague neuromuscular changes (such as tremor), vague GI symptoms (such as nausea), and slow, weak pulse

a liter of fluid. Body fluids contain two types of solutes: electrolytes, which dissociate into charged particles (or ions), and a number of substances that don't dissociate into ions — glucose, creatinine, and urea, for example. Although the ICF and ECF contain different solutes, the overall concentrations of the two fluids are essentially equal.

Osmolarity refers to the number of osmols, the standard unit of osmotic pressure, per liter of solution. It's expressed as milliosmols per liter (mOsm/liter). Sometimes you'll hear the term *osmolality* used interchangeably with osmolarity. But they're not exactly the same. Osmolality refers to the number of osmols per kilogram of solution

Understanding body fluid distribution

Body fluid is distributed between two main compartments—intracellular and extracellular. Extracellular fluid itself has two components—interstitial fluid and plasma. This illustration shows body fluid distribution for an adult.

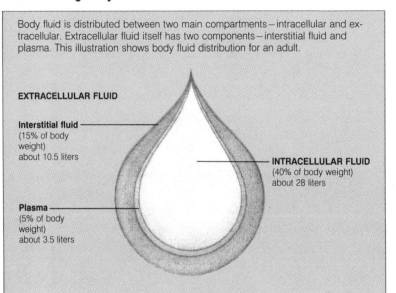

EXTRACELLULAR FLUID

Interstitial fluid
(15% of body
weight)
about 10.5 liters

Plasma
(5% of body
weight)
about 3.5 liters

INTRACELLULAR FLUID
(40% of body weight)
about 28 liters

and is expressed as mOsm/kg. Because most calculations of body fluid solute concentrations are based on osmolarity, you'll find that term used in this book. Both ICF and ECF have an osmolarity of about 300 mOsm/liter.

Fluid and solute movement
The constant movement of fluid and solutes between body fluid compartments maintains fluid and electrolyte balance. This movement involves several different processes. Solutes move between compartments mainly by diffusion and active transport; fluid moves by osmosis and capillary dynamics. Membrane permeability and hydrostatic and osmotic pressures influence these movement processes.

Diffusion. Most solutes move by diffusion; that is, they go from an area of higher concentration to one of lower concentration. This is known as moving down the concentration gradient. The result is an equal distribution of solutes. Because diffusion requires no energy, it's considered a form of passive transport.

Active transport. By contrast, active transport involves physiologic pumps that move solutes from an area of lower concentration to one of higher concentration. You'll hear this referred to as moving against the gradient.

Active transport requires adenosine triphosphate for energy; production of this high-energy molecule depends on oxygen and glucose availability. You're probably familiar with one active transport pump—the sodium-potassium pump. It moves sodium ions from inside the cell to the ECF and potassium ions in the opposite direction. Other examples of solutes actively transported across cell membranes include calcium ions, hydrogen ions, several sugars, and amino acids.

Osmosis. When two areas with different concentrations are separated by a membrane that allows fluid but not solutes to pass, the fluid moves by osmosis. It flows passively across the membrane from the area of low solute concentration to the area of high solute concentration. This dilution process stops when the solute concentrations on both sides of the membrane are equal.

Fluid moves by osmosis between the ECF and the ICF according to the osmolarity of the compartments. Normally, the osmotic pressures of the ECF and ICF are equal. If the osmolarity of the ECF increases, water will shift by osmosis from the ICF into the ECF. Conversely, if the ICF osmolarity increases, water will shift from the ECF into the ICF.

Keep in mind that osmosis can create a fluid imbalance — unequal fluid volumes in the ECF and ICF compartments despite equal concentrations of solute. This can produce serious complications.

Capillary dynamics. If the osmotic pressure inside and outside the cells is the same, as it normally is, no *net* water movement occurs. But water must leave the plasma, circulate past cells, and pick up waste products. The water and dissolved wastes then have to reenter the plasma and circulate to the kidneys so the waste can be excreted and water volume adjusted. This water movement occurs continuously by means of capillary filtration and reabsorption.

Within the vascular system, only the capillaries have walls thin enough to let solutes pass. Capillary filtration results from hydrostatic (or fluid) pressure and blood pressure against the walls of the capillary. When the blood pressure inside the capillary exceeds the fluid pressure outside, it forces fluid and solutes out through the capillary-wall pores and into the ISF.

If no force opposed capillary filtration, plasma would move in only one direction — out of the capillaries. Obviously, that would lead to severe hypovolemia and shock. Fortunately, during filtration, albumin (a protein that can't pass through capillary walls) remains behind in a diminishing volume of water. As albumin concentration inside the capillaries increases, albumin begins to draw water back in by osmosis. This process, called reabsorption, opposes filtration, making it possible for water to return to the capillaries. The osmotic, or pulling, force of albumin is referred to as colloid osmotic pressure (COP) or oncotic pressure. It averages 25 mm Hg through the entire capillary.

As long as capillary blood pressure exceeds COP, water and diffusible solutes can leave the capillaries and circulate into the ISF. When capillary blood pressure falls below COP, water and diffusible solutes return to the capillaries. Normally, in any capillary, blood pressure exceeds COP up to the vessel's midpoint, then falls below COP along the rest of the vessel. So capillary filtration occurs along the capillary's first half, and reabsorption occurs along the second half. And, as long as capillary blood pressure and plasma albumin levels remain normal, no net movement of water occurs. Occasionally, a slight net filtration does occur. When this happens, the excess fluid moves passively into the lymphatic vessels located just outside the capillaries around the cells. This fluid eventually returns to the right atrium.

Fluid and electrolyte regulation

Each day, of course, the body gains and loses fluid. For the body to maintain fluid volume and concentration, the gains must equal the losses (see *Daily fluid gains and losses,* page 12). This balancing act involves the kidneys, heart, liver, adrenal and pituitary glands, nervous system, and certain hormones.

Basically, regulation of fluid volume and concentration depends on the interaction of two hormones: antidiuretic hormone (ADH), which acts to retain water, and aldosterone, which acts to retain sodium. The thirst mechanism helps make these hormones effective.

Antidiuretic hormone. Produced in the hypothalamus, ADH is stored in and released from the posterior pituitary gland. The hormone responds to osmolarity and to blood pressure changes (which normally reflect blood volume changes). Increased serum osmolarity stimulates ADH release, which, in turn, promotes renal reabsorption of water. The result: excretion of concentrated urine. Conversely, decreased serum osmolarity inhibits ADH release, reducing renal reabsorption of water. In this case, diuresis results.

This hormone can also correct a loss of blood volume, even if osmolarity isn't affected. As you may know, atrial receptors sensitive to pressure (or stretch) are connected by nerve axons to the hypothalamus and posterior pituitary gland. Normally, the pressure of blood on these receptors triggers nerve impulses that inhibit the production and release of ADH. With declining atrial blood pressure, stimulation of the receptors decreases. Thus, ADH production and release intensify, causing the kidneys to reabsorb more water. In this way, blood volume can increase and blood pressure can return to normal.

ADH doesn't do all this alone. Remember, fluid balance and electrolyte balance are interdependent. As water is reabsorbed to increase blood volume, osmotically active particles must be added to prevent fluid dilution. The hormone aldosterone makes this possible, but only after a complex series of steps involving the kidneys, liver, and adrenal gland.

Aldosterone. Secreted by the adrenal cortex, this hormone regulates sodium reabsorption. Aldosterone initiates the active transport of sodium into the blood in the distal convoluted tubules and collecting ducts of the kidneys. Because sodium is the major osmotically active solute in ECF, aldosterone can maintain appropriate osmolarity as fluid volume expands to compensate for diminished blood volume.

Here's how aldosterone secretion occurs. As blood volume declines, blood flow and blood pressure at the renal glomeruli decrease. This triggers the kidneys to release the hormone renin into the blood. As renin circulates, it encounters the inactive protein angiotensinogen, which is continuously produced by the liver. Renin converts angiotensinogen to an active form, angiotensin I. This then converts to angiotensin II, which stimulates the adrenal cortex to secrete aldosterone and begin counteracting the fall in blood volume.

Daily fluid gains and losses

Each day the body gains and loses fluid through several different processes. The illustration below shows the main sites involved. The amounts shown apply to adults; infants exchange a greater amount of fluid than adults.

Note: Gastric, intestinal, pancreatic, and biliary secretions total about 8,200 ml, but these are almost completely reabsorbed, so they're not usually counted in daily fluid gains and losses.

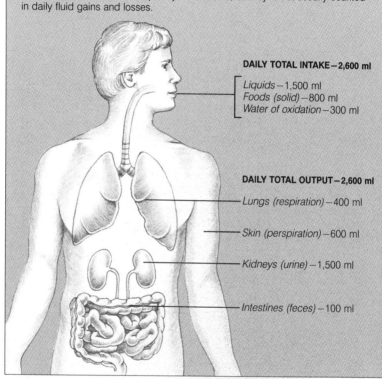

DAILY TOTAL INTAKE—2,600 ml

Liquids—1,500 ml
Foods (solid)—800 ml
Water of oxidation—300 ml

DAILY TOTAL OUTPUT—2,600 ml

Lungs (respiration)—400 ml

Skin (perspiration)—600 ml

Kidneys (urine)—1,500 ml

Intestines (feces)—100 ml

Thirst mechanism. As mentioned, this mechanism helps make ADH and aldosterone effective. Here's how. When a person is thirsty, he drinks more fluid. And the ingested fluid is absorbed from the intestine into the plasma. From the plasma, fluid can move freely between fluid compartments, diluting solute concentrations and promoting osmolarity as needed.

What makes a person thirsty in the first place? Increased ECF osmolarity (from loss of body water or intake of highly salty foods, for example) stimulates the thirst center in the hypothalamus. So when the thirst mechanism works normally, it helps maintain fluid and electrolyte balance. Keep in mind, however, that in elderly people, the thirst mechanism usually becomes less effective, making them prone to dehydration.

Understanding the types of I.V. solutions

Solutions used for I.V. therapy may be isotonic, hypotonic, or hypertonic. Which type you give a patient depends on whether you want to change or maintain his body fluid status.

Isotonic solution	**Hypotonic solution**	**Hypertonic solution**
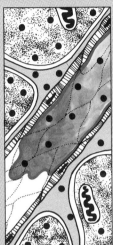	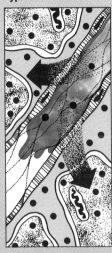	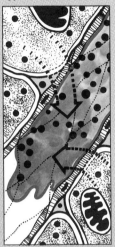
An *isotonic* solution has an osmolarity about equal to that of serum. It expands the intravascular and interstitial compartments.	A *hypotonic* solution has an osmolarity lower than that of serum. It shifts fluid and electrolytes out of the intravascular compartment, hydrating the intracellular and interstitial compartments.	A *hypertonic* solution has an osmolarity higher than that of serum. It draws fluid and electrolytes into the intravascular compartment from the intracellular and interstitial compartments.

I.V. solutions

The effect an I.V. solution has on the fluid compartments depends on how the solution's osmolarity compares with the patient's serum osmolarity. Normally, serum has the same osmolarity as other body fluids, about 300 mOsm/l. A lower serum osmolarity suggests fluid overload; a higher osmolarity suggests hemoconcentration and dehydration. For a particular patient, the doctor will choose an I.V. solution that will maintain or restore fluid balance. He can chose from three basic types: isotonic, hypotonic, and hypertonic solutions (see *Understanding the types of I.V. solutions*, and *Quick guide to I.V. solutions*, page 14).

Isotonic solutions. An isotonic I.V. solution possesses the same osmolarity (or tonicity) as serum and

Quick guide to I.V. solutions

A solution is isotonic if its osmolarity falls within (or near) the normal range for serum (275 to 295 mOsm/liter). A hypotonic solution has a lower osmolarity; a hypertonic solution, a higher one.

This chart lists common examples of the three types of I.V. solutions and provides key considerations for administering them.

SOLUTION	EXAMPLES	NURSING CONSIDERATIONS
Isotonic *[handwritten: FOR: Hypotension]*	• Lactated Ringer's (275 mOsm/liter) • Ringer's (275 mOsm/liter) • 0.9% sodium chloride (normal saline) (308 mOsm/liter) • D₅W (260 mOsm/liter)	• Because these solutions expand the intravascular and interstitial compartments, closely monitor your patient for signs of fluid overload – especially if he has hypertension or congestive heart failure. • Because the liver converts lactate to bicarbonate, don't give lactated Ringer's solution if the patient's blood pH exceeds 7.5. • Don't give lactated Ringer's solution if the patient has liver disease because he won't be able to metabolize lactate. • Avoid giving D₅W to a patient at risk for increased intracranial pressure (ICP), because it acts like a hypotonic solution. (Although usually considered isotonic, D₅W is actually isotonic only in the container. After administration, dextrose is quickly metabolized, leaving only water – a hypotonic fluid.)
Hypotonic *[handwritten: → dehydration from diuretic use → hyperglycemia → hyperosmolar nonketonic syndrome]*	• 0.45% saline (154 mOsm/liter) • 0.33% saline (103 mOsm/liter) • dextrose 2.5% in water (126 mOsm/liter)	• Administer cautiously. These solutions can cause a sudden fluid shift from blood vessels into cells. This could cause cardiovascular collapse from intravascular fluid depletion and increased ICP from fluid shift into brain cells. • Don't give hypotonic solutions to patients at risk for increased ICP from cerebrovascular accident, head trauma, or neurosurgery. • Don't give hypotonic solutions to patients at risk for third-space fluid shifts (abnormal fluid shifts into the interstitial compartment or a body cavity) – for example, patients suffering from burns, trauma, or low serum protein levels from malnutrition or liver disease.
Hypertonic *[handwritten: can irritate veins]* *[handwritten: → post-op to: stabilize BP, maintain urine output, reduce edema]*	• dextrose 5% in 0.45% saline (406 mOsm/liter) • dextrose 5% in normal saline (560 mOsm/liter) • dextrose 5% in lactated Ringer's (575 mOsm/liter)	• Because these solutions greatly expand the intravascular compartment, closely monitor your patient for circulatory overload. • Hypertonic solutions pull fluid from the intracellular compartment, so don't give them to a patient with a condition that causes cellular dehydration – for example, diabetic ketoacidosis. • Don't give hypertonic solutions to a patient with impaired heart or kidney function – his system can't handle the extra fluid.

ther body fluids. Because this type of solution doesn't alter serum osmolarity, it stays within the intravascular compartment and the interstitial compartment. The solution expands these compartments without pulling fluid from the intracellular compartment.

One indication for an isotonic solution would be hypotension from hypovolemia. Common isotonic solutions include lactated Ringer's and normal saline. Usually, you'd give an isotonic solution through a peripheral vein.

Hypotonic solutions. A hypotonic I.V. solution has an osmolarity lower than that of serum. When a patient receives this type of solution, his body fluid and electrolytes shift out of the blood vessels and into the cells and interstitial spaces, where osmolarity is higher. So a hypotonic solution hydrates cells while depleting the circulatory system.

Hypotonic solutions may be called for when diuretic therapy dehydrates body cells. Other indications include hyperglycemic conditions, such as diabetic ketoacidosis and hyperosmolar nonketotic syndrome. In these conditions, high serum glucose levels draw fluid out of cells.

Hypertonic solutions. A hypertonic I.V. solution has a higher osmolarity than serum. When a patient receives this type of solution, fluid and electrolytes are pulled from the intracellular and interstitial compartments into the intravascular compartment, raising serum osmolarity.

You may see hypertonic solutions ordered for some patients postoperatively. That's because the shift of fluid into the blood vessels reduces the risk of edema, stabilizes blood pressure, and helps maintain urine output. When you give these solutions, keep in mind that they may irritate the veins.

Administration advice

So far, we've reviewed what I.V. therapy is and why it's used. We've also discussed the basic physiologic principles that govern its use. Now let's turn to two key areas of administering I.V. therapy: controlling infection and maintaining flow rates.

Infection control

Infection control measures protect your patient and you. Your patient runs a high risk of infection just because he needs I.V. therapy. And whenever you're exposed to blood and body fluids, you're at risk for hepatitis B virus (HBV) and human immunodeficiency virus (HIV).

Protecting your patient. A patient may be exposed to infection because of poor skin preparation, improper manufacturing or storage of equipment, or a break in aseptic technique — to name just a few potential dangers. To reduce his risk of I.V.-related infection, follow these guidelines:
- Wash your hands before touching or manipulating any I.V. equipment or fluids and before starting an I.V. infusion.
- Clip hairs at the venipuncture site.
- Clean the venipuncture site with an approved antiseptic. The Intravenous Nurses Society (INS) recommends cleaning with 70% isopropyl alcohol or povidone-iodine solution, then applying iodophor ointment or another microbial agent after the site dries.
- Check the I.V. equipment before using it. This includes checking

solutions for particulate matter and noting the expiration dates on packages.
- Never reuse a catheter or needle.
- Always cover the venipuncture site with a sterile dressing and change the dressing as recommended by INS standards—that is, every 48 hours and whenever soiled, wet, or loose.
- Change I.V. administration sets as recommended by hospital policy and whenever you note or suspect a break in aseptic technique. The INS recommends changing administration sets every 48 hours in most situations (preferably when adding a new container of I.V. solution) and I.V. catheters every 48 to 72 hours (preferably every 48 hours).

Sometimes, despite all these precautions, infection still develops. If you detect an infection at the venipuncture site, take these steps:
- Culture any drainage before removing the I.V. catheter.
- Remove the catheter carefully, holding it by the hub and not touching any part that was under the patient's skin.
- Use sterile scissors to cut the catheter just below the hub, allowing the part that was under the skin to drop into a sterile container. Cover the container with a sterile cap. Label it and send it to the laboratory to be cultured.
- Label the container of I.V. fluid and send it to the laboratory for a culture.
- Record the lot numbers of all equipment.

After taking these steps, you can resume I.V. therapy, but you must use all new sterile equipment and change the site. If at all possible, use the patient's other arm.

Protecting yourself. When performing I.V. therapy, follow the univer-sal precautions developed by the Centers for Disease Control (CDC) for persons who perform invasive procedures. The CDC recommends that blood and body fluids from *all* patients be treated as potentially infected with HBV or HIV, which are both blood-borne viruses. You should pay special attention to the precautions on proper handling of needles and sharp instruments and the use of barriers.
- Use disposable needles whenever possible. Place once-used needles in a puncture-resistant container as quickly as possible.
- To prevent needle-stick injuries, don't bend or break needles, recap them, separate them from the syringe, or in any way manipulate them by hand.
- Wear gloves whenever you work with I.V. infusions and equipment. Discard the gloves in the appropriate waste receptacle after each use.
- Wash your hands before and after working with I.V. equipment. Wash your hands immediately if they come in contact with blood or other body fluids.
- If you foresee any possibility of blood or body fluid splashing or splattering, wear additional appropriate forms of barrier protection, such as a gown, a mask, and eye protection.

As an adjunct to its universal precautions, the CDC recommends that you be immunized with the HBV vaccine.

I.V. flow rates
When carrying out I.V. therapy, you must maintain accurate flow rates for the prescribed solutions. If an infusion runs too fast or too slow, your patient may suffer complications, such as phlebitis, loss of venous patency, infiltration, circulatory overload (possibly leading to

ongestive heart failure and pulmo-
ary edema), and adverse drug
reactions. To prevent such complica-
ons, you need to correctly calcu-
ate the I.V. flow rate from the
doctor's order and then regulate it.
For more information, see *Compo-
ents of an I.V. order.)*

Calculating the flow rate. When you
regulate the I.V. flow rate with a
lamp or a controller, the rate will
usually be measured in drops/
minute. (If you use a volumetric
pump instead, the flow rate will be
measured in ml/hour.)

I.V. administration sets deliver a
specific number of drops per milliliter. You'll find this number on the
package label of the set. Standard
macrodrip sets deliver 10 to 20
drops/ml, depending on the manufacturer; microdrip sets deliver
60 drops/ml; and blood transfusion
sets deliver 10 drops/ml. An adapter
can convert a macrodrip set to a
microdrip system.

To calculate the drip rate, use the
formula provided in *Calculating
flow rates*, pages 18 and 19. After
determining the desired drip rate,
remove your watch or position your
wrist so you can look at your watch
and the drops at the same time.
Then adjust the clamp to achieve
the approximate drip rate, and
count the drops for 1 minute. Readjust the clamp, as necessary, and
count the drops for another minute.
Keep adjusting the clamp and counting the drops until you have the
correct rate.

Regulating the flow rate. You can
regulate the I.V. flow rate with two
types of clamps — the screw clamp
and the roller clamp. The screw
clamp gives you greater accuracy.
But you'll find the roller clamp, used
for standard fluid therapy, faster

Components of an I.V. order

Orders for I.V. therapy may be stan-
dardized for different illnesses and
therapies (such as burn treatment) or
individualized for a particular patient.
Some hospital policies dictate an au-
tomatic stop-order for I.V. fluids. For
example, I.V. orders are good for 24
hours from the time they're written, unless otherwise specified.

A complete order for I.V. therapy
should specify the following:
• type and amount of solution
• any additives and their concentrations (such as 10 mEq potassium
chloride in 500 ml dextrose 5% in
water).
• rate or volume of infusion
• duration of infusion.

If you find that an order isn't complete, consult the doctor. You should
also consult him if you think the order
is inappropriate because of the patient's condition.

and easier to manipulate. A third
type, the slide clamp, can stop
or start the flow but can't regulate
the rate (see *Using I.V. clamps,*
page 20).

Typically, you'll also use another
type of flow control device, called
a rate minder, which will be added
to the I.V. tubing. You can set
this device to the desired flow rate,
then label it to indicate the rate in
ml/hour. Rate minders do have some
limitations. They provide accurate
flow only with certain venipuncture
devices in place — usually 20G or
larger. And rate minders don't
usually deliver infusions at rates
lower than 5 to 10 ml/hour. For this
reason, they're used mainly in
adult patients.

When you're depending on a
clamp, you have to monitor the flow
rate closely and adjust it as needed.

ates

...y the flow rate of I.V. solu... ...ber that the number of drops requi...d to deliver 1 ml varies with the type of administration set used and the manufacturer. The illustration at top right shows a standard (macrodrip) set, which delivers from 10 to 20 drops/ml. The illustration in the center shows a pediatric (microdrip) set, which delivers about 60 drops/ml. The illustration at bottom right shows a blood transfusion set, which delivers about 10 drops/ml.

To calculate the flow rate, you must know the calibration of the drip rate for each manufacturer's product. As a quick guide, refer to the chart below. Use this formula to calculate specific drip rates:

$$\frac{\text{Volume of infusion (in ml)}}{\text{time of infusion (in minutes)}} \times \text{drop factor (in drops/ml)} = \text{drops/minute}$$

		ORDERED VOLUME					
		500 ml/ 24 hr or 21 ml/hr	1,000 ml/24 hr or 42 ml/hr	1,000 ml/20 hr or 50 ml/hr	1,000 ml/10 hr or 100 ml/hr	1,000 ml/8 hr or 125 ml/hr	1,000 ml/6 hr or 166 ml/hr
ADMINISTRA-TION SET	DROPS/ML	DROPS/MINUTE TO INFUSE					
Macrodrip Abbott	15	5	10	12	25	31	42
Baxter Healthcare	10	3	7	8	17	21	28
Cutter	20	7	14	17	34	42	56
IVAC	20	7	14	17	34	42	56
McGaw	15	5	10	12	25	31	42
Microdrip Various manufacturers	60	21	42	50	100	125	166

Such factors as venous spasm, venous pressure changes, patient movement, manipulations of the clamp, and bent or kinked tubing can cause the rate to vary markedly. You can easily monitor the flow rate by using a time tape, which marks the prescribed solution level at hourly intervals (see *Using a time tape,* page 21).

Usually, if the patient's condition requires that precise rates be main-

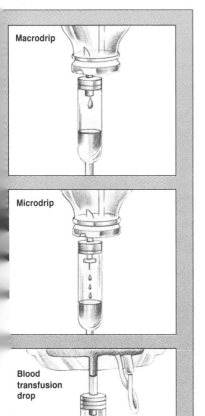

Macrodrip

Microdrip

Blood transfusion drop

Factors affecting the flow rate.
Besides the flow control clamp, several factors can affect the I.V. flow rate: the type of I.V. fluid, the height of the I.V. container, the type of administration set, and the size, thickness, and position of the venipuncture device.

• *Infused fluids.* Thick or viscous fluids such as blood products, colloids such as albumin, suspensions such as amphotericin B, and highly osmolar solutions may be difficult to infuse. You can dilute these solutions with compatible fluid, or you can administer them using an infusion control device to maintain the correct flow rate. With an admixture such as an antibiotic solution, you must completely dilute the drug when reconstituting it, then agitate the container. This ensures a uniform solution, aids the flow, and prevents a bolus effect. When giving blood products, such as red blood cells and platelets, you'll have to *gently* agitate the container during the infusion because denser cells tend to clump on the bottom.

• *Container height.* The type of I.V. solution container doesn't usually affect the flow rate, but the height of the container does. Always hang the I.V. container far enough above the patient's heart to overcome his normal blood pressure. Usually, about 36″ (91 cm) between the peripheral I.V. site and the container will do. For a CV line, you may have to hang the container higher or use an infusion control device to overcome the higher venous pressure.

• *Administration sets.* You'll see many different types of gravity control sets. Some are straight drip sets (usually macrodrip at 10, 15, or 20 drops/ml); some are volume-control sets (usually microdrip at 60 drops/ml). For most adult patients,

ained, you should use an infusion ontrol device, such as an I.V. pump r controller. These devices help revent significant changes in the fusion rate. If possible, use such a evice when infusing medications.

EQUIPMENT

 Using I.V. clamps

You may use a roller or a screw clamp to regulate the flow of an I.V. solution. With these clamps, you use a wheel or screw to increase and decrease the flow through the I.V. line. The slide clamp moves horizontally to open and close the I.V. line. It can stop and start the flow but doesn't allow fine adjustments to regulate the flow. (Arrows indicate the direction you turn or push to open the clamp.)

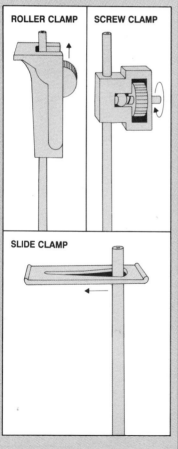

ROLLER CLAMP **SCREW CLAMP**

SLIDE CLAMP

you'll find that a macrodrip set is accurate enough to maintain infusions. However, fluid viscosity may alter the drop size, creating slight changes in the volume delivered. Microdrip sets, which you'll use for pediatric patients, deliver fluid at a more accurate rate because drop size doesn't vary significantly.

If the I.V. therapy requires an evacuated glass container, use a vented set. Otherwise, the flow rate will be hampered because air can't get into the bottle to displace the fluid. With bags of fluid, you can use either vented or nonvented sets.

• *Type of venipuncture device.* The diameter of the venipuncture device as well as the vein size also affect flow rate. The devices vary in size from the narrowest butterfly needle (27G) to the widest plastic I.V. catheter (14G). As you'd expect, the narrower the venipuncture device, the slower the infusion. To protect your patient, always choose the narrowest venipuncture device possible for the size of the vein and the viscosity of the solution.

Remember, thin-walled, narrow-gauge venipuncture devices allow flow rates comparable to thicker-walled, wide-gauge venipuncture devices. (Even blood products and colloids can be infused through 24G thin-walled devices without damage.) For pediatric and elderly patients, use infusion control devices with narrow-gauge catheters.

The position of the venipuncture device will also affect the flow rate. If the opening is against the wall of the vein or near a valve, the flow may diminish or even stop.

Checking the flow rate. Check your patient's I.V. flow rate according to your hospital's policy. How often you check the rate depends on several factors, including the pa-ient's condition and age as well as he I.V. solution. Many nurses check he flow rate every time they're in a patient's room and after each position change. You should check he flow rate more often when caring for intensive care patients, pediatric patients, and patients who are receiving a drug that can cause damage if extravasation occurs.

With each check, inspect the I.V. site for complications and assess the patient's response to the therapy. Determine the flow rate by counting he number of drops/minute, as you did when setting the rate initially. For potentially toxic infusions, be sure to time the flow for a full minute to ensure accuracy.

If the infusion rate slows significantly, you can usually get it back on schedule by adjusting the rate slightly. Don't make a major adjustment, though. If the rate must be increased more than 30%, consult he doctor. If the flow has stopped, see *What to do when an infusion stops,* pages 22 and 23.

You should also time an infusion control device or rate minder once per shift. (These devices have an error rate ranging from 2% to 10%.) Before using any infusion control device, become thoroughly familiar with its features. Obtain in-service instruction and perform return demonstrations until you learn the system. (For more information, see *Infusion control devices: When the alarm goes off,* page 24.)

Legal and patient-care issues

Now that we've covered some specific I.V. therapy procedures, we'll
Text continues on page 24.)

Using a time tape

Here's a simple way to monitor the I.V. flow rate. Attach a piece of tape or a preprinted strip to the I.V. container. Then write hourly times on the tape or strip beginning with the time you hung the solution.

By comparing the actual time with the label time, you can quickly see if the rate needs to be adjusted. Remember that you should never increase I.V. rates more than 30% unless you consult with the doctor.

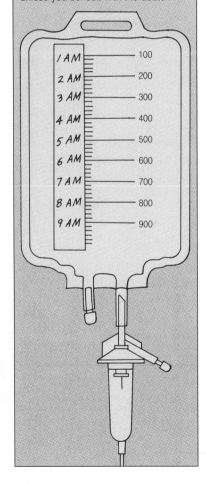

What to do when an infusion stops

When an infusion stops, systematically assess the I.V. system from the patient to the fluid container, looking for potential trouble areas.

Check the I.V. site (1)
Check for infiltration or phlebitis, which may slow or stop the flow rate.

Check for patency (2)
Evaluate the I.V. device for patency, which may be affected by several factors.
• If the patient's limb is flexed or lying directly on the I.V. site, increased blood pressure may stop the flow. Reposition the limb as necessary.
• The tip of the needle may be against the vein wall or a venous valve. Lift up or pull back the venipuncture device to reestablish the I.V. flow.
• If the patient's arm is wrapped with tape, a tourniquet effect may reduce the flow rate. Taping the I.V. site too tightly can cause the same problem. Release or remove tape. Then reapply it.
• Smaller venipuncture devices may kink or fold, impeding I.V. flow. Pull the device back to reestablish flow.
• Local edema or poor tissue perfusion from disease may block venous flow. Move the I.V. line to an unaffected site.
• Infusion of incompatible fluids or medications may cause a precipitate to form. This can block the I.V. tubing and venipuncture device, and may even expose the patient to a life-threatening embolism. Always check the compatibility of medications and I.V. solutions before administration. Replace the venipuncture device if it's occluded.

Check the filter (3)
Make sure the in-line filter is the right size and type. I.V. fluids are usually run through a 0.22- or 0.45-micron filter that eliminates air and microorganisms from the system. Single-use filters shouldn't be used for in-line filtration—only for drawing up a medication or administering a bolus dose.

If you use the wrong size or type of filter, the solution may not pass through it. For example, drugs such as amphotericin B and lymphocyte immune globulin (Atgam) consist of molecules too large to pass through a 0.22-micron filter; they'd rapidly block the filter and stop the I.V. flow. If necessary, replace the filter.

A filter that's used longer than recommended may become blocked by minute particles and microorganisms. Not only will the I.V. flow stop, but the patient may become exposed to bacterial toxins and sepsis. The interval between filter changes usually ranges from 24 to 48 hours, depending on the manufacturer's instructions. Change the filter if necessary.

Check clamps (4)
Be sure that the flow clamps are open. Check all clamps, including the roller clamp and any clamps on secondary sets, such as a slide clamp on a filter. (A roller clamp may also become jammed if the roller is pushed up too far.)

Check tubing (5)
Determine if the tubing is kinked or if the patient is lying on it. Also check whether the tubing remains crimped where a clamp was tightened around it. If so, gently squeezing the area between your fingers will usually round out the tubing to its original shape.

Check air vents (6)
If you're using an evacuated glass container, you need an air vent to make the solution flow. Insert one as necessary. With a volume-control set, an air vent is

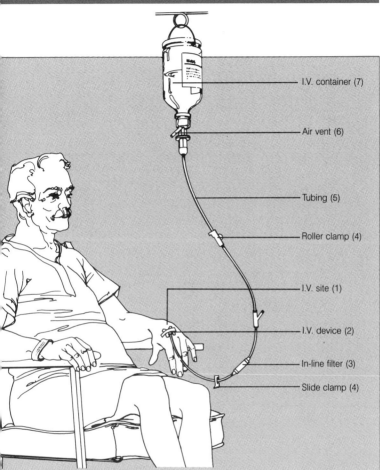

I.V. container (7)

Air vent (6)

Tubing (5)

Roller clamp (4)

I.V. site (1)

I.V. device (2)

In-line filter (3)

Slide clamp (4)

usually located at the top of the calibrated chamber. If the solution flow stops, check the patency of this vent and the position of the vent clamp. To check patency, follow the manufacturer's instructions.

Check fluid level (7)
Observe the fluid level in the I.V. container. If it's empty, replace it as ordered. If the solution is cold, it may be causing venous spasm and thus decreasing the flow rate. Applying warm compresses may relieve venous spasm and help increase the flow rate. Make sure subsequent solutions are at room temperature. Finally, check to see if the spike at the end of the administration set has been pushed far enough into the container to allow the solution to flow.

If you can't identify the problem with this series of checks, the I.V. line should be removed and restarted at a different site. Be sure to document the episode in the patient's chart.

TROUBLESHOOTING

 Infusion control devices: When the alarm goes off

When the alarm on an infusion control device goes off, check for the following.	
Air in the line	While setting up, make sure all air is out of the line, including air trapped in Y sites. Also, check that the connections are secure and the container is filled properly. Withdraw any air from a piggyback port with a syringe or an air-eliminating filter. A wet-air detector may give a false reading.
Infusion completed	Reset the pump as ordered or discontinue the infusion. A slow keep-vein-open flow rate will usually keep the I.V. line patent as long as enough fluid remains.
Empty container	Check for adequate fluid levels in the I.V. container and have another container available before the last one runs out.
Low battery	Battery life varies; keep the machine plugged in on AC power as much as possible, especially while the patient is in bed. If the alarm goes off, plug in the machine immediately, or power may be lost for a while (usually a half hour to several hours).
Occlusion	Check that all clamps are open, look for kinked tubing, and check the patency of the venipuncture device.
Rate change	Check that the infusion control device displays the ordered rate. The patient or a family member may have tampered with the controls.
Open door	The door should be closed; it may not shut if the device isn't set up properly (for example, if the cassette isn't inserted all the way).
Malfunction	A mechanical failure usually must be handled by the biomedical engineering department or the manufacturer. Disconnect the infusion control device. Label it clearly with a *broken* sign and indicate the specific problem.

look at four key areas: legal implications of I.V. therapy, documentation, patient teaching, and home care.

Legal implications
Nurses now participate in complex I.V. therapy procedures that were once performed only by doctors. Because of this change, questions exist about your legal right to give I.V. therapy. Of course, such legal uncertainty can be intimidating—especially because any violation of the Medical Practice Act is a crimi-

al offense. To protect yourself, you must know the legal basis for nursing practice in I.V. therapy and the functions you can legally perform in the state where you work. The legal basis for nursing practice in I.V. therapy is determined by state nurse practice acts, joint policy statements, and institutional policy. All three provide you with legal protection as long as you act correctly and within the limitations they set up.

State nurse practice acts. Each state has such an act, defining the duties a nurse may or may not perform. These acts serve as guidelines and place limits on nursing practice.

Joint policy statements. These position papers also serve as guidelines and place limits on nursing practice. State nurses' associations and at least two other organizations (such as the state medical society and the state hospital association) develop these statements, which require that nurses be held liable for their knowledge, skill, and judgment. According to these statements, you may refuse to perform an I.V. therapy procedure if, in your judgment, you're not qualified or competent. For example, if you've never been taught venipuncture, you may refuse to carry out the procedure until you receive proper education. The law won't excuse negligence because you carry out a doctor's order.

Institutional policy. Every health care institution has I.V. therapy policies that determine which duties you may and may not perform. These policies can't go beyond what the state nurse practice act and joint policy statements permit, but they may further limit your duties.

In short, these policies serve as the final word on what you can and can't do.

The INS has developed standards for practice in I.V. therapy. In many cases, committees that develop institutional policy use these standards. But remember, INS standards serve only as guidelines. The committees responsible for developing institutional policy aren't required to follow INS standards.

Documentation

You need to document I.V. therapy for a couple of reasons. For one thing, an accurate description of your care provides legal protection. For another, good documentation furnishes health care insurers with the record they need of the equipment and supplies used.

You may document I.V. therapy on progress notes, a special I.V. therapy sheet or flow sheet, or a nursing care plan on the patient's chart. You also have to document it on the intake and output sheet.

Starting I.V. therapy. When documenting the insertion of a venipuncture device or the beginning of therapy, specify the following:
• size and type of device
• name of the person who inserted the device
• date and time
• I.V. site
• type of solution
• any additives
• flow rate
• use of any electronic infusion device
• complications, patient response, and nursing interventions
• patient teaching and evidence of patient understanding (for example, ability to explain instructions or perform a return demonstration).

At the insertion site, you should

also have a label with the size and type of the device, the name of the person who inserted it, and the date and time it was inserted.

Maintaining I.V. therapy. When documenting I.V. therapy maintenance, specify the following:
• condition of site
• site care
• dressing changes
• site changes
• tubing and solution changes
• patient teaching and evidence of patient understanding.

If you obtain a specimen and send it to the laboratory for culture and sensitivity testing, document your actions along with the name of the doctor who ordered the test.

Number each container sequentially over the course of I.V. therapy. For example, if 3,000 ml of solution is ordered on May 10, you'd number that day's 1,000-ml bottles as 1, 2, 3. If another 3,000 ml is ordered on May 11, you'd number those bottles as 4, 5, 6. This system helps reduce administration errors.

If you're using an I.V. flow chart, record the date, flow rate, use of any electronic flow device, type of solution, and sequential solution container number. Also, note the date and time of dressing and tubing changes.

Discontinuing I.V. therapy. When documenting the discontinuation of I.V. therapy, be sure to specify the following:
• time and date
• reason for discontinuing therapy
• patient reactions, complications, and nursing interventions
• follow-up actions (for example, applying a bandage to the site or restarting the I.V. infusion in another limb).

Intake and output sheet. When you're documenting I.V. therapy on the intake and output sheet, follow these guidelines:
• If the patient is a child, note fluid levels on the I.V. bottles and bags hourly. If the patient is an adult, note these levels at least twice a shift.
• With children and certain critical-care patients, record intake of all I.V. infusions, including fluids, medications, flush solutions, blood and blood products, and TPN every hour.
• Document the total amount of each infusate, as well as grand totals of all infusions (including piggybacks), so you can monitor fluid balance.
• Also note output, either hourly or less often, depending on the patient's needs. Output includes urine, stool, vomitus, and GI drainage.
• Read fluid levels from the glass container, plastic container (you may need to pull the bag taut for a more accurate reading), or volume-control set. These levels can give you an estimate of the amounts infused and the amounts remaining to be infused.

Labels. Whenever you place a new dressing over an I.V. site, you must label it. Note the date and time of the insertion and the type and size of the needle or catheter on pieces of tape. Write your initials on the last piece of tape (see *How to label a dressing,*).

You should also label the I.V. fluid container and, as discussed earlier, place a time tape on it. With a child, you may label the volume-control set, instead of the container. Your label should include the following:
• patient's name, identification number, and room number
• date and time the container was hung

- any additives, including dosages
- sequential container number
- expiration date and time of the infusion
- your name.

Patient teaching

Although I.V. therapy may be a common treatment to health care professionals, it probably isn't to your patient. He may be apprehensive about the procedure and concerned that his condition has worsened. If your patient is a child, his fears may be completely unrealistic. He may think he's about to be poisoned or that the needle will never be removed. So you need to help your patient relax. Try to take the mystery out of I.V. therapy by teaching him and, when appropriate, his family about it.

Information and assurance. Begin by assessing your patient's previous experience, his expectations, and his knowledge of venipuncture and I.V. therapy. Then base your teaching on this assessment. You can use pamphlets, sample catheters and I.V. equipment, slides, and videotapes as well as any appropriate information provided by other patients. Be sure to explain why your patient needs I.V. therapy, how venipuncture is performed, how I.V. therapy will limit his activities, and how he can help maintain the proper flow rate.

Allow him to express his concerns and fears. Of course, you'll reassure him, but you can also help by encouraging him to use stress-reduction techniques such as deep, slow breathing. Also allow the patient and his family to participate in his care as much as possible.

Evaluating your teaching. You should evaluate how well your pa-

How to label a dressing

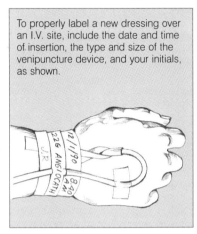

To properly label a new dressing over an I.V. site, include the date and time of insertion, the type and size of the venipuncture device, and your initials, as shown.

tient and his family understand your instruction while you're teaching and when you're done. You can do this by asking frequent questions and by having them explain or demonstrate what you've taught.

Document all your teaching in the patient's records. Note what you taught and how well the patient understood it.

Home I.V. therapy

More and more, patients are receiving I.V. therapy at home. Such home therapy benefits both patients and hospitals. Patients feel more comfortable in their homes, and they're able to perform many of their normal activities. Plus, I.V. therapy at home costs less — for the patient and the hospital.

Types of therapy. A home care patient may receive fluids, antibiotics, antifungals, chemotherapeutic agents, insulin, chelating agents, or medications for pain control. More recently, some blood products have been given at home following an an initial infusion in the hospital.

The patient can use several types of preparations:
• I.V. drip medications mixed in 50- or 100-ml minibags that can be refrigerated or frozen
• I.V. push medications that can be mixed and administered
• medications for external or implanted pumps
• blood components for bleeding disorders
• special premixed infusions that can be injected through a collapsible balloon reservoir at the I.V. site.

Patient selection. Candidates for home I.V. therapy must be selected carefully. A home care patient must be willing and able to learn how to administer I.V. therapy safely. He also must learn the potential complications and interventions and understand asepsis. And he must be able to order necessary supplies.

If he needs help, the patient must have a home caregiver—typically a family member or friend. His home should allow him to administer I.V. therapy safely and conveniently. And, obviously, he must have the financial resources to cover the cost of therapy.

Teaching the home care patient. Instruction for home I.V. therapy usually begins in the hospital with a demonstration and discussion of the appropriate procedures. Your patient and his home caregiver must be able to demonstrate the procedures successfully and answer your questions satisfactorily before the patient can be discharged.

Also, before discharge, make sure that the patient has a skilled nursing service for home I.V. therapy. He'll also need to contact a company that distributes the necessary supplies. Some companies have a 24-hour hot line to deal with patient problems regarding equipment and supplies. Ideally, the company should be close enough to deliver. If the patient is going to need supplies while traveling, advise him to contact a national company.

If blood studies must be done during therapy, make arrangements for a nurse to go to the patient's home to draw blood or for the patient to go to a laboratory. If the patient will need general nursing services other than I.V. therapy services, contact a home care nursing agency. Finally, be certain that your patient and his family understand everything they must do to administer I.V. therapy safely and efficiently at home.

Suggested readings

Delaney, C.W., and Lauer, M. *Intravenous Therapy: A Guide to Quality Care.* Philadelphia: J.B. Lippincott Co., 1988.

Gasparis, L., et al. "I.V. Solutions: Which One's Right for Your Patient?" *Nursing89* 19(4):62-64, April 1989.

LaRocca, J.C. *Pocket Guide to Intravenous Therapy.* St. Louis: C.V. Mosby Co., 1989.

Metabolic Problems. NurseReview Series Springhouse, Pa.: Springhouse Corp., 1988.

Nursing91 I.V. Drug Handbook. Springhouse, Pa.: Springhouse Corp., 1991.

Plumer, A.L., and Cosentino, F. *Principles and Practice of Intravenous Therapy,* 4th ed. Boston: Little, Brown & Co., 1987.

2

PERIPHERAL I.V. THERAPY

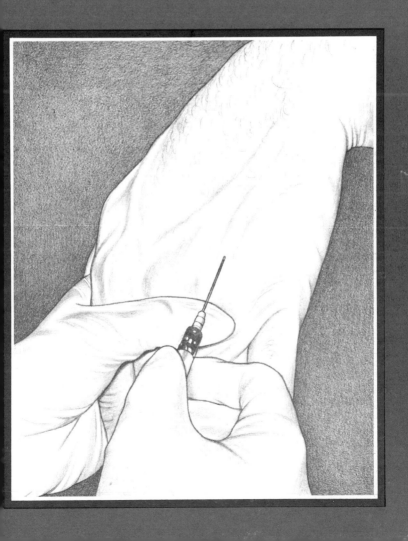

Few nursing responsibilities require more time, knowledge, and skill than administering peripheral I.V. therapy. At the patient's bedside, you need to assemble the equipment, prepare the patient, insert the venipuncture device, regulate the I.V. flow rate, and monitor the patient for adverse effects. You also have certain "behind-the-scenes" responsibilities, such as checking the doctor's orders, ordering supplies, labeling solutions and tubings, and documenting your nursing interventions.

Perhaps the most challenging aspect of peripheral I.V. therapy is performing the venipuncture itself. The procedure requires good motor skills and the ability to recognize and correct problems. Becoming proficient at venipuncture takes time and practice, but it's worth the effort. As you gain experience, you'll learn to perform even difficult venipunctures confidently and successfully, decreasing your patient's anxiety and discomfort. Expert venipuncture skills also help prevent extravasation, a common complication of peripheral I.V. therapy.

This chapter will help you acquire and refine your peripheral I.V. skills by explaining how to prepare for and perform a venipuncture. The chapter will also tell you how to maintain and discontinue peripheral infusions. But first comes a quick overview of peripheral I.V. therapy.

Basics of peripheral I.V. therapy

Peripheral I.V. therapy may be ordered whenever venous access is needed—for example, when a patient requires surgery, transfusion therapy, or emergency care. You may use peripheral I.V. therapy to maintain hydration, to restore fluid and electrolyte balance, to provide fluids for resuscitation, or to administer I.V. drugs, blood and blood components, or nutrient solutions for metabolic support.

Advantages and disadvantages
Peripheral I.V. therapy offers several advantages, including easy access to veins and rapid administration of solutions, blood, and drugs. This therapy also allows continuous administration of drugs and brings about rapid systemic changes. Plus, the administration sites are easy to see and thus to monitor.

As with any invasive vascular procedure, peripheral I.V. therapy carries associated risks, such as infection and bleeding. Also, the rapid administration of some I.V. drugs can produce irreversible adverse effects, such as hearing loss, bone marrow depression, or kidney or heart damage. And peripheral I.V. therapy can be used only for a limited amount of time. Finally, although peripheral I.V. therapy is less expensive than other invasive vascular procedures, it's still more costly than oral, S.C., or I.M. administration.

Preparing for venipuncture and infusion

Before performing a venipuncture, you need to prepare your patient by teaching him what to expect and by helping him relax. You also need to select the proper equipment

Antibiotic Prophylaxis for Endoscopic Procedures

PATIENT CONDITION	PROCEDURE CONTEMPLATED	ANTIBIOTIC PROPHYLAXIS
High risk: Prosthetic Valve Hx Endocarditis Syst-Pulm Shunt Synth Vasc Graft (<1yr old) Complex Cyanotic congenital heart disease	Stricture Dilation Variceal Sclerotherapy ERCP/obstructed biliary tree	Recommended
	Other endoscopic procedures including EGD and colonoscopy (with or without biopsy/polypectomy), variceal ligation	Prophylaxis optional
Moderate Risk: Most other congenital abnormalities Acquired valvular dysfunction (e.g. rheumatic heart disease) Hypertrophic Cardiomyopathy Mitral valve prolapse with regurgitation or thickened leaflets	Esophageal Stricture Dilation Variceal Sclerotherapy	Prophylaxis optional
	Other endoscopic procedures including EGD and colonoscopy (with or without biopsy/polypectomy), variceal ligation	Not recommended
Low Risk: Other cardiac conditions (CABG, repaired septal defect or patent ductus, mitral valve prolapse without valvular regurgitation, isolated secundum atrial septal defect, physiologic/functional/innocent heart murmurs, rheumatic fever without valvular dysfunction, pacemakers, implantable defibrillators)	All endoscopic procedures	Not recommended
bstructed bile duct	ERCP	Recommended
ancreatic cystic lesion	ERCP, EUS-FNA	Recommended
rrhosis acute GI bleed	All endoscopic procedures	Recommended
scites, Immunocompromised tient	Stricture Dilation Variceal Sclerotherapy	No recommendation
	Other endoscopic procedures including EGD and colonoscopy (with or without biopsy/polypectomy), variceal ligation	Not recommended
patients	Percutaneous endoscopic feeding tube placement	Recommended (parenteral cephalosporin or equivalent)
thetic joints	All endoscopic procedures	Not recommended

ac Prophylaxis Regimens (oral 1 hour before, IM or IV 30 mins before procedure)
xicillin PO or Ampicillin IV: adult 2.0 g, child 50 mg/kg Penicillin allergic: Clindamycin
t 600 mg, child 20 mg/kg), OR Cephalexin OR cefadroxil (adults 2.0 g, child 50 mg/kg), OR
romycin OR clarithromycin (adult 500 mg, child 15 mg/kg), OR Cefazolin (adult 1.0 g , child
g/kg IV or IM), OR Vancomycin (Adult 1.0 g, child 10-20 mg/kg IV)

American Society for Gastrointestinal Endoscopy
1520 Kensington Road, Suite 202, Oak Brook, IL 60523
(P) 630-573-0600 (F) 630-573-0691
E-mail: info@asge.org   Web site: www.asge.org

The Management of Anticoagulants and Anti-Inflammatory Medications in Patients Undergoing Endoscopic Procedures

PROCEDURE RISK	Condition Risk for Thromboembolism	
	HIGH	LOW
HIGH	Discontinue warfarin 3-5 days before procedure. Consider heparin while INR is below therapeutic level.	Discontinue warfarin 3-5 days before procedure. Reinstitute warfarin after procedure.
LOW	No change in anticoagulation. Elective procedures should be delayed while INR is in supratherapeutic range.	

PROCEDURE RISK

High Risk Procedures	*Low Risk Procedures*

• Polypectomy
• Biliary Sphincterotomy
• Pneumatic or bougie dilation
• PEG placement
• Endosonographic guided fine needle aspiration
• Laser ablation and coagulation
• Treatment of varices
	• Diagnostic
	   EGD ± biopsy
	   Flex sig ± biopsy
	• ERCP without sphincterotomy
	• Biliary/pancreatic stent without endoscopic sphincterotomy
	• Endosonography without fine needle aspiration
	• Enteroscopy

CONDITION RISK

High Risk Procedures	*Low Risk Procedures*
• Atrial fibrillation associated with valvular heart disease • Mechanical valve in the mitral position • Mechanical valve and prior thromboembolic event	• Deep vein thrombosis • Uncomplicated or paroxysmal nonvalvular atrial fibrillation • Bioprosthetic valve • Mechanical valve in the aortic position

Aspirin and Other NSAID Use

In the absence of a pre-existing bleeding disorder, endoscopic procedures may be performed in patients taking aspirin or other NSAIDS.

MAY

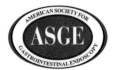

American Society for Gastrointestinal Endoscopy
1520 Kensington Road, Suite 202, Oak Brook, IL 60523
(P) 630-573-0600 (F) 630-573-0691
E-mail: info@asge.org   Web site: www.asge.org

Teaching your patient about I.V. therapy

Many patients feel apprehensive about peripheral I.V. therapy. So before you begin therapy, teach your patient what to expect before, during, and after the procedure. Thorough patient teaching can reduce his anxiety, making therapy easier. Follow these guidelines:

☐ Describe the procedure to the patient. Tell him that "intravenous" means inside the vein and that a plastic catheter or needle will be placed in his vein. Explain that fluids containing certain nutrients or medications will flow from an I.V. bag or bottle through a length of tubing, then through the plastic catheter or needle into his vein.

☐ Tell the patient approximately how long the catheter or needle will stay in place. Explain that the doctor will decide how much and what type of fluid he needs.

☐ Mention that he may feel transient pain during insertion but that the discomfort will stop once the catheter or needle is in place.

☐ Tell him the I.V. fluid may feel cold at first. Reassure him that this should last only a few minutes.

☐ Tell him to report any discomfort after the catheter or needle has been inserted and the fluid has begun to flow.

☐ Explain any restrictions, as ordered. If appropriate, tell the patient he can walk while receiving I.V. therapy. Depending on the insertion site and the device, he may also be able to shower or take a tub bath during therapy.

☐ Teach the patient how to care for the I.V. line. Tell him not to pull at the insertion site or tubing and not to remove the container from the I.V. pole. Also, tell him not to kink the tubing or lie on it. Explain that he should call a nurse if the flow rate suddenly slows down or speeds up.

☐ Explain that removing a peripheral I.V. line is a simple procedure. Tell the patient that pressure will be applied to the site until the bleeding stops. Reassure him that once the device is out and the bleeding stops, he'll be able to use his arm or leg normally.

and prepare it for use. Then you must choose the best possible venipuncture site and device for the patient's needs.

Preparing the patient

Begin by checking the patient's medical record for allergies. Then review the doctor's orders and note any pertinent laboratory studies.

Many patients, especially those who've never had peripheral I.V. therapy, will be apprehensive. And this apprehension can cause vasoconstriction, making the venipuncture more difficult for you and more painful for the patient. You can help decrease your patient's anxiety by preparing him for therapy.

Careful patient teaching and a confident, understanding attitude will help your patient relax and cooperate during the procedure. (See *Teaching your patient about I.V. therapy.*)

When you meet the patient, greet him by name and introduce yourself. Explain what you're about to do in simple, understandable terms, and tell him that he can help by relaxing and remaining as still as possible during the procedure. If the patient seems extremely anxious, suggest that he slowly inhale and exhale to help decrease his anxiety. Reassure him that you'll make the procedure as quick and painless as possible.

EQUIPMENT

Comparing I.V. administration sets

I.V. administration sets come in three major types: basic, add-a-line, and volume-control. The basic set is used to administer most I.V. solutions. An add-a-line set delivers an intermittent secondary infusion through one or more additional Y-sites. A volume-control set delivers small, precise amounts of solution. All three types come with vented or nonvented drip chambers, depending on the type of solution container being used. (Glass containers require a vented drip chamber; plastic containers don't.)

BASIC SET　　　　　　　　　　　　　　　　**ADD-A-LINE SET**

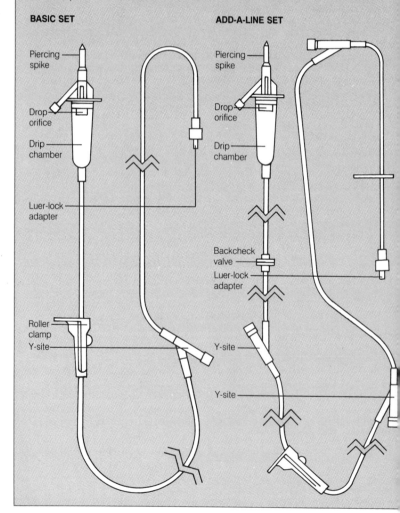

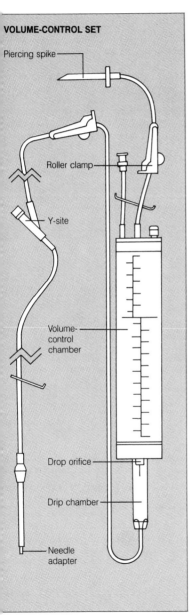

VOLUME-CONTROL SET

Piercing spike

Roller clamp

Y-site

Volume-control chamber

Drop orifice

Drip chamber

Needle adapter

Provide privacy by asking visitors to leave and by drawing the curtains around the bed if another patient is present. Give the patient a gown if he isn't already wearing one, and have him remove any jewelry from the arm where the I.V. site will be. Position him comfortably in the bed, preferably on his back. Make sure that the area is well lit and that the bed is at the proper height for the procedure.

Selecting the equipment

Besides the venipuncture device, peripheral I.V. therapy requires a solution container, an administration set, an in-line filter (if ordered), and, if needed, an infusion pump or controller.

Solution containers. Two basic types of I.V. solution containers exist: glass and plastic. Although plastic bags are widely used for routine administration of I.V. fluids, sterile glass bottles must be used to deliver medications that are absorbed by plastic — diazepam and insulin, for example. Also, some hospitals routinely use glass bottles.

Glass I.V. containers form part of either a closed system or an open system. Because these bottles are evacuated, they quickly pull in injected additives. A vented I.V. administration set balances the outflow of fluid and provides sufficient air intake to enable the solution to flow correctly. (Vented administration sets have an extra filtered port near the spike to allow air entry.) In a closed system, only filtered air is admitted to the container. In an open system, unfiltered air enters the bottle through a plastic tube in the container.

Available in soft, flexible bags or semirigid rectangular containers, plastic I.V. containers allow easy

EQUIPMENT

Supplemental I.V. equipment

When administering I.V. therapy, you may use certain additional pieces of equipment — including extension tubing, I.V. loops, T-connectors, and flow regulators. Before attaching this equipment to the venipuncture device, you must purge the tubing of air.

Extension tubing
Extending 6″ to 12″ (15 to 30 cm), this small-bore tubing can be attached to any I.V. tubing. Unlike large-bore tubing, it allows a smaller loop tubing to adjoin the venipuncture device. It also allows I.V. tubing to be changed away from the insertion site, thereby reducing the risk of contamination.

I.V. loop
Shaped like a small horseshoe and made of small-bore tubing, an I.V. loop connector fits between the venipuncture device and I.V. tubing. It enables the tubing to be changed away from the device and facilitates stabilization of the device.

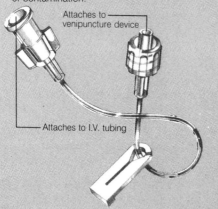

Attaches to venipuncture device

Attaches to I.V. tubing

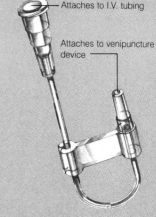

Attaches to I.V. tubing

Attaches to venipuncture device

storage, transport, and disposal. Unlike glass bottles, plastic containers are nonevacuated: They collapse as fluid flows out and don't require air venting, thereby reducing the risk of air embolism or airborne contamination.

Administration sets. You'll see three major types of I.V. administration sets — basic, add-a-line, and volume-control. (See *Comparing I.V. administration sets,* pages 32 and 33.) Depending on the type of therapy, you may also need supplemental equipment, such as a flow regulator, a T-connector, an I.V. loop, and extension tubing. (See *Supplemental I.V. equipment.*)

Selection of the set depends on the rate and type of infusion and the type of solution container. When selecting an administration set, be sure you know the flow rate the set is gauged to produce. Also, consider the nature of the I.V. solution: The more viscous the solution, the larger the drops, and thus the fewer drops per milliliter.

Administration sets come with

T-connector

Useful for simultaneous administration of fluids and drugs, this small-bore extension tubing is 3" to 6" (7.5 to 15 cm) long and has an injection site near its luer-lock adapter. You'll attach the luer end to the venipuncture device and the opposite end to the I.V. tubing. Then another I.V. needle can be inserted into the latex injection cap. This added injection site can also serve as an intermittent infusion device — for example, a heparin lock — while the primary I.V. solution infuses. This device often eliminates the need for insertion of a second venipuncture device.

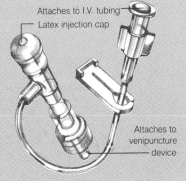

Attaches to I.V. tubing
Latex injection cap

Attaches to venipuncture device

Flow regulator

By delivering a spec... ...milliliters per hour, flow reg... ...elp ensure accurate delivery o... ...v. fluids. Although not as accurate as infusion pumps or controllers, flow regulators are most reliable with inactive patients.

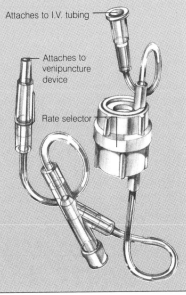

Attaches to I.V. tubing

Attaches to venipuncture device

Rate selector

two types of drip systems — macrodrip and microdrip. A macrodrip set delivers a solution in large quantities at rapid rates. A microdrip set delivers a smaller amount of solution with each drop. It's used for pediatric patients and for adults requiring small or closely regulated amounts of I.V. solution.

• *Basic sets*. A basic I.V. administration set consists of a piercing spike, a drop orifice, a drip chamber, one or more Y-site injection ports, a roller clamp, and a luer-lock adapter or needle adapter. Basic sets range from

70" to 110" (178 to 279 cm) long and can be vented or nonvented. They're used to deliver any I.V. solution or to infuse solutions through a heparin lock. A secondary injection port permits separate or simultaneous infusion of two solutions.

Depending on the size of the drop orifice, a basic set will deliver 10, 15, or 20 gtt/ml. Basic sets are also available with microdrip systems, which deliver 60 gtt/ml (or 60 ml/hour).

• *Add-a-line sets*. When a patient needs an intermittent secondary

add-a-line administra-
can deliver the solution
ough one or more additional Y-
sites. A special valve located on the
set — commonly called the backcheck valve — prevents backflow of
the secondary solution into the
primary solution. After the secondary solution has been infused, the
set automatically resumes infusing
the primary one.

• *Volume-control sets.* Used primarily for pediatric patients, this set
delivers small, precise amounts of
fluids and medications from a volume-control chamber. Calibrated in
milliliters, this chamber is placed
at the top of the I.V. tubing just
above the drip chamber. Also called
burette sets, these sets are available
with or without an in-line filter and
may be attached directly to the
venipuncture device or connected as
a secondary infusion into a Y-site
of a primary I.V. administration set.
Macrodrip and microdrip systems
are available.

In-line filters. Located in the fluid
pathway between the I.V. tubing
and the venipuncture device, in-line
filters remove pathogens and particles, thus reducing the risk of infection and phlebitis. Filters also help
prevent air from entering a patient's
circulation by venting it through
the filter housing.

Filters range in size from 0.22
micron (the most common) to 170
microns. Some filters are built into
the line; others need to be added.
Although the Intravenous Nurses
Society (INS) recommends routine
use of a 0.22-micron final in-line
filter, most hospitals establish their
own policies on size.

Certain filters are made only for
use with gravity flow; if the pressure exceeds a certain level, the
filter may crack. So when you use a
filter with an infusion pump, make
sure it can withstand the pump's
pressure.

Carefully prime an in-line filter to
eliminate all the air from it, following the manufacturer's directions.

Usually, you can expect to use an
in-line filter:
• for an immunosuppressed patient
• when administering total parenteral nutrition
• when using additives composed of
many separate particles (such as
antibiotics that require reconstitution) or when administering several
additives
• when the risk of phlebitis is high.

Avoid using an in-line filter when
administering solutions with large
particles that can clog the filter — for
example, suspensions (such as amphotericin B), emulsions (such as
Liposyn), and high-molecular-vol-
ume plasma expanders (such as
dextran). Also avoid filters when
administering 5 mg or less of a drug
because the filter may absorb it.

Be sure to change the filter when
the manufacturer recommends.
This helps prevent bacteria from
accumulating and releasing endo-
toxins and pyrogens small enough to
pass through the filter into the
bloodstream. Also, remember that
filters merely complement I.V.
therapy; they don't replace the need
for strict aseptic technique.

Controllers and pumps. These electronically controlled infusion devices
deliver I.V. solutions more accurately than other devices. Used for
both central venous and peripheral
I.V. therapy, infusion controllers
and pumps deliver solutions with
95% to 98% accuracy and indicate
when the infusion is completed.
They also save valuable time by detecting infusion problems, such as
air in the line, low batteries, ma-

chine malfunctions, occlusion, and inability to deliver at the set rate. Depending on the problem, the device may shut off, sound or flash an alarm, or switch to a keep-vein-open rate. (See *Regulating flow rate electronically,* page 38.)

• *I.V. controllers.* Placed about 36″ (91 cm) above the I.V. site, an I.V. controller regulates gravity flow by counting drops of infused solution with a photoelectronic eye. The device monitors the flow rate and indicates rate changes with an alarm. The alarm also helps detect infiltration — for instance, when back pressure from infiltrated fluid slows the flow rate.

Relatively inexpensive, controllers work well with uncomplicated infusions for adults. They're less likely to cause complications than I.V. pumps. However, they're less accurate than pumps because they merely count drops instead of measuring the flow rate in ml/hour. Moreover, position changes commonly trigger false alarms.

• *I.V. infusion pumps.* These devices apply pressure to the infusion to maintain the preset flow rate. You'll find pumps especially useful when administering viscous solutions or using small-gauge venipuncture devices. Infusion pumps also help when patient activity increases venous back pressure.

Infusion pumps come in many sizes and types. Some models can administer piggyback solutions; others can administer from 2 to 10 infusions simultaneously.

Infusion pumps save you time by eliminating the need for counting drops and adjusting flow rates. Pumps also offer key safety benefits. For instance, the controlled flow rate reduces the risk of circulatory overload. And because the pressure generated by the pump exceeds the maximum venous pressure, any increase in venous pressure caused by coughing, crying, or straining won't change the flow rate. Some models also reduce the risk of air embolism by sounding an alarm or stopping the infusion when the I.V. container is empty.

Despite their advantages, infusion pumps do have some drawbacks. They're more expensive to use than I.V. controllers. Plus, the pressure they exert increases the risk of undetected infiltration.

Peristaltic action pumps apply pressure to the I.V. tubing to force the solution through it. These pumps are easy to prime, but most aren't recommended for delicate fluids that might break down under pressure — blood cells, for example.

Piston-cylinder pumps come in two basic models: syringe and volumetric. Both types infuse a specific volume of fluid, using a small plunger. With a syringe pump, you place a prefilled syringe in the chamber and set the rate. A pump then pushes the plunger forward, delivering the I.V. solution. Portable and compact, syringe pumps are used for small doses. They're ideal for home care, for administering fluids to infants, and for delivering intra-arterial drugs.

In a volumetric pump, a disposable cassette pulls fluid from a container and delivers it at a certain rate over a specific period. Most volumetric pumps operate at moderate pressures (up to 15 psi) and can deliver 1 to 999 ml/hour with 97% to 98% accuracy.

You may also see certain specialized pumps and infusers — such as an ambulatory patient-controlled analgesia (PCA) infusion pump, which can deliver intermittent doses, a continuous infusion, or doses on demand.

EQUIPMENT

Regulating flow rate electronically

Controllers and infusion pumps, such as the two shown below, electronically regulate the flow of I.V. solutions and drugs. You'll use them when a precise flow rate is required—for instance, when administering total parenteral nutrition solutions and chemotherapeutic or cardiovascular agents.

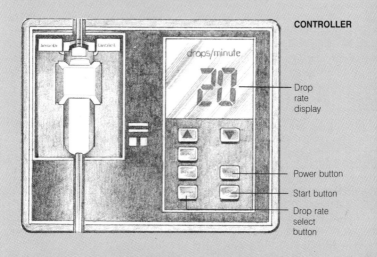

CONTROLLER

Drop rate display

Power button

Start button

Drop rate select button

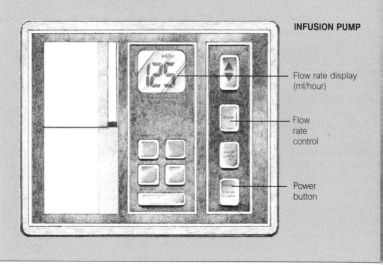

INFUSION PUMP

Flow rate display (ml/hour)

Flow rate control

Power button

Preparing the equipment

After you've selected and gathered the infusion equipment, you need to prepare it for use. This involves inspecting the I.V. container and solution, preparing the solution, attaching and priming the administration set, and setting up the controller or infusion pump.

Inspecting the container and solution. Check that the container size and the type of infusate are correct. Note the expiration date; discard an outdated solution.

Make sure that the solution container is intact. Examine a glass container for cracks or chips, or a plastic container for tears or leaks. (Plastic bags often come with an outer wrapper, which you must remove before inspecting the container.) Small cracks or leaks may admit microorganisms, so be sure to discard a damaged container, even if the solution appears clear. If the solution isn't clear, discard it and notify the pharmacy or dispensing department. Solutions may vary in color, but they should never appear cloudy, turbid, or separated.

Finally, inspect the container's cap to make sure it's intact. If the pharmacist has instilled additives into the I.V. container, the cap may have been resealed.

Preparing the solution. Using sterile technique, remove the cap from a glass container or the plastic pull tab from a plastic container. Be careful not to contaminate the port. Then label the container with the following information: your name; the patient's name, identification number, and room number; the date and time the container was hung; any additives; and the container number. With pediatric patients, you may label the volume-control set

instead of the container.

Attaching the administration set.
Choose an administration set that's correct for the patient and the type of I.V. container and solution you're using. Examine the set for cracks, holes, and missing clamps. Then prepare the solution container and attach it to the administration set.
• *Preparing a nonvented bottle.*
If necessary, remove the metal cap and inner disk. Place the bottle on a stable surface and wipe the rubber stopper with an alcohol swab. Close the flow clamp on the administration set.

Then remove the protective cap from the administration set spike and push the spike through the center of the rubber stopper. Avoid twisting or angling the spike to prevent pieces of the stopper from breaking off and falling into the solution.

Now invert the bottle. If the vacuum is intact, you'll hear a hissing sound and see air bubbles rising. (This may not happen if a medication has been added to the bottle.) If the vacuum isn't intact, discard the bottle. If it is, hang the bottle on the I.V. pole, about 36″ (91 cm) above the venipuncture site.
• *Preparing a vented bottle.* Remove the bottle's metal cap and latex diaphragm to release the vacuum. If the vacuum isn't intact, discard the bottle (unless a medication has been added). Place the bottle on a stable surface and wipe the rubber stopper with an alcohol swab. Close the flow clamp.

Now remove the protective cap from the administration set spike. Push the spike through the insertion port, which is located next to the air vent. Hang the bottle on the I.V. pole about 36″ above the venipuncture site.

• *Preparing a plastic bag.* Place the bag on a flat, stable surface or hang it on an I.V. pole. Then remove the protective cap or tear the tab from the tubing insertion port. Slide the flow clamp on the administration set up close to the drip chamber and close the clamp.

Remove the protective cap from the administration set spike. Holding the port carefully and firmly with one hand, quickly insert the spike with your other hand. Hang the bag about 36″ above the venipuncture site.

Priming the administration set.

Label the administration set with the date and time you opened it. Be sure you've labeled the container, as mentioned before.

• *Priming a basic set.* First, squeeze the drip chamber until it's half full. Then, aim the distal end of the tubing at a receptacle. (Most distal tube coverings allow the solution to flow without having to remove the protective end.) Now open the roller clamp and allow the solution to flow through the tubing to remove air. Close the clamp after the solution has run through the line and all air bubbles are purged.

• *Priming an add-a-line set.* Follow the same steps you'd use to prime a basic set, along with these additional steps. As the solution flows through the tubing, tap the back-check valve to release trapped air bubbles. Then straighten the tubing and continue purging air in the usual manner.

• *Priming a volume-control set.* Attach the set to the solution container and close the lower clamp on the I.V. tubing. Open the clamp between the solution container and the fluid chamber, and allow about 50 ml of the solution to flow into the chamber. Close the upper clamp.

Now open the lower clamp and allow the solution in the chamber to flow through the remainder of the tubing. Make sure that some fluid remains in the chamber so that air won't fill the tubing below it. Close the lower clamp. Then fill the chamber with the desired amount of solution.

If you're using a filter on any of these sets, attach it to the primed distal end of the I.V. tubing and follow the manufacturer's instructions for filling and priming it. Most filters are positioned with the distal end of the tubing facing upward so that the solution will completely wet the filter membrane and all air bubbles will be eliminated from the line.

Setting up a controller or an infusion pump.
First, attach the controller or pump to the I.V. pole. Then, insert the administration spike into the I.V. container.

If you're using a controller, fill the drip chamber no more than halfway; otherwise, the device may miscount the drops. Rotate the chamber so the fluid touches all sides; this removes any vapor that could interfere with counting drops. If you're using a pump, fill the drip chamber completely to prevent air bubbles from entering the tubing.

Now follow the manufacturer's instructions for priming the tubing and for placing the drop sensor and the I.V. tubing (if you're using a controller) or just the I.V. tubing (if you're using an infusion pump).

Place the controller or pump on the same side of the bed as the I.V. setup or the intended venipuncture site. Set the appropriate controls on the machine to the desired infusion rate or volume. Check the patency of the I.V. line and watch for infiltration. If you're using a controller, monitor the accuracy of the infusion rate.

Turn on the alarm switches. Be sure to explain the alarm system to the patient, so he isn't frightened when a change in the infusion rate triggers the alarm.

Frequently check the controller or pump to make sure it's working properly—specifically, note the flow rate. Monitor the patient for signs of infiltration and other complications, such as infection and air embolism. (See *Preventing problems with infusion pumps.*) Change the tubing according to the manufacturer's instructions or hospital policy.

Selecting the insertion site

Successful I.V. therapy depends on selecting the best possible venipuncture site. When choosing a site, consider the vein's location and condition, the purpose of the infusion, the duration of the therapy, the cooperation needed by the patient and, when possible, the patient's preference.

Usually, you select a vein in the nondominant arm or hand. Never select a vein in an edematous or impaired arm or leg. Consider accessibility, but keep in mind the most prominent vein isn't necessarily the best choice. It may have sclerosis or be in an unsuitable location.

Perform subsequent venipunctures proximal to a previously used or injured vein. Be sure to rotate access sites. (See *Identifying peripheral venipuncture sites,* page 42.)

Commonly used veins. The veins commonly used for placement of venipuncture devices include the metacarpal, cephalic, and basilic along with the branches that extend from them. (See *Comparing peripheral venipuncture sites,* pages 43

CHECKLIST

Preventing problems with infusion pumps

An infusion pump can be a valuable tool. It saves time and helps ensure your patient's safety. But you still need to monitor the patient for complications, such as infiltration and infection. You also need to check the pump itself to make sure it's working properly.

You can avoid several common infusion pump problems by following this advice:

☐ Follow the manufacturer's instructions precisely when you insert the tubing. *Note:* To avoid fluid overload, clamp the tubing when the pump door is open.

☐ Be sure to flush *all* air out of the tubing before connecting it to the patient; this lowers the risk of air embolism.

☐ Double-check the flow rate. The control setting may not be accurate. Monitor the flow rate over a specific time span, then adjust the flow as needed.

☐ Avoid turning the pump on and off excessively. This can clog the catheter.

☐ Before you attach an I.V. filter or infuse blood, check the manufacturer's recommendations. Not all pumps are designed for these purposes.

and 44.) Veins of the hand and forearm are suitable for most drugs and solutions. The cephalic and basilic veins in the upper arms are more suitable for irritating drugs and solutions with a high osmolarity. The saphenous vein of the inner aspect of the ankle and the veins of the dorsal network are best when leg or foot veins must be used.

In most cases, a venipuncture device placed in an upper arm vein will be comfortable and less likely

(Text continues on page 44.)

Identifying peripheral venipuncture sites

Where are the best venipuncture sites? Generally, the superficial veins in the dorsum of the hand and the forearm offer the most choices. The dorsum of the hand is well supplied with small, superficial veins that can be dilated easily and usually accommodate either a needle or a catheter. In the forearm, the basilic, cephalic, and median antebrachial veins have fairly large diameters—plus they're long and straight. Thus, they make convenient sites for introducing the large-bore needles and longer I.V. catheters used in prolonged I.V. therapy. When trauma renders these sites impractical, the feet and legs provide acceptable secondary choices for venipuncture. In infants under age 6 months, scalp veins are frequently used.

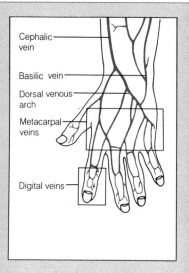

Cephalic vein
Basilic vein
Dorsal venous arch
Metacarpal veins
Digital veins

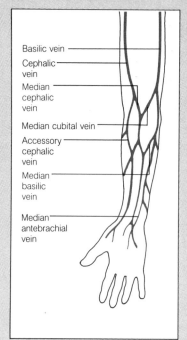

Basilic vein
Cephalic vein
Median cephalic vein
Median cubital vein
Accessory cephalic vein
Median basilic vein
Median antebrachial vein

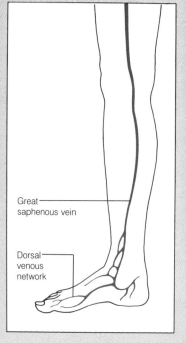

Great saphenous vein
Dorsal venous network

Comparing peripheral venipuncture sites

Venipuncture sites located in the hand, the forearm, and the foot and leg offer various advantages and disadvantages. The following chart includes some of the major benefits and drawbacks of several common venipuncture sites.

SITE	ADVANTAGES	DISADVANTAGES
Digital veins Run along lateral and dorsal portions of fingers	• May be used for short-term therapy. • May be used when other means aren't available.	• Fingers must be splinted with a tongue blade, decreasing ability to use hand. • Uncomfortable for patient. • Infiltration occurs easily. • Can't be used if veins in dorsum of hand already used.
Metacarpal veins On dorsum of hand; formed by union of digital veins between knuckles	• Easily accessible. • Lie flat on back of hand. • In adult or large child, bones of hand act as splint.	• Wrist movement decreased unless a short catheter is used. • Insertion more painful because more nerve endings in hands. • Site becomes phlebitic more easily.
Accessory cephalic vein Runs along radial bone as a continuation of metacarpal veins of thumb	• Large vein excellent for venipuncture. • Readily accepts large-gauge needles. • Doesn't impair mobility. • Doesn't require an armboard in an older child or adult.	• Sometimes difficult to position catheter flush with skin. • Usually uncomfortable. Venipuncture device at bend of wrist, so movement causes discomfort.
Cephalic vein Runs along radial side of forearm and upper arm	• Large vein excellent for venipuncture. • Readily accepts large-gauge needles. • Doesn't impair mobility.	• Proximity to elbow may decrease joint movement. • Vein tends to roll during insertion.
Median antebrachial vein Arises from palm and runs along ulnar side of forearm	• Vein holds winged needles well. • A last resort when no other means are available.	• Many nerve endings in area may cause painful venipuncture or suffer infiltration damage. • Infiltration occurs easily in this area.
Basilic vein Runs along ulnar side of forearm and upper arm	• Will take a large-gauge needle easily. • Straight strong vein suitable for large-gauge venipuncture devices.	• Uncomfortable position for patient during insertion. • Penetration of dermal layer of skin where nerve endings are located causes pain. • Vein tends to roll during insertion.

(continued)

Comparing peripheral venipuncture sites *(continued)*

SITE	ADVANTAGES	DISADVANTAGES
Antecubital veins Located in antecubital fossa (median cephalic, located on radial side; median basilic, on ulnar side; median cubital rises in front of elbow joint)	• Large veins facilitate drawing blood. • Often visible or palpable in children when other veins won't dilate. • May be used in an emergency or as a last resort.	• Difficult to splint elbow area with armboard. • Median cephalic vein crosses in front of brachial artery. • Veins may be small and scarred if blood has been drawn frequently from this site.
Great saphenous vein Located at internal malleolus	• Large vein excellent for venipuncture.	• Circulation of lower leg may be impaired. • Walking difficult with device in place. • Increased risk of deep vein thrombosis.
Dorsal venous network Located on dorsal portion of foot	• Suitable for infants and toddlers.	• Vein may be difficult to see or find if edema is present. • Walking difficult with device in place. • Increased risk of deep vein thrombosis.

to be pulled out accidentally. Thus, such a vein is a good choice when the device must stay in place longer than usual. But the upper arm veins have some serious drawbacks. When an upper arm vein has an I.V. device in place, you can't use the lower veins in that arm. Moreover, upper arm veins can be difficult to locate in obese patients or in those with short arms.

Before choosing a vein as an I.V. site, make sure it's actually a vein — not an artery. Located deep in the muscles, arteries contain bright red blood that flows away from the heart. A single artery supplies a large area. If you puncture an artery, blood will pulsate from the site. Conversely, veins are superficial and contain dark red blood that flows toward the heart. Many veins supply the same area. If you puncture a vein, the blood flows

slowly from the site. (See *Reviewing anatomy of the skin and veins*, pages 46 and 47.)

All major veins have valves, but they're usually apparent only in long, straight arm veins or in patients with large, well-developed veins. You should avoid having the tip of the venipuncture device terminate in a valve because this position could affect the flow rate.

Selection guidelines. When selecting an I.V. site, choose distal veins first, unless the solution is very irritating (for example, 40 mEq or more of potassium chloride). Any peripheral vein is usable; today, even the digital veins are sometimes used. But to decrease discomfort, you should choose a vein that's full, soft, and long. It should be large enough to allow blood flow around the catheter; this will minimize venous irritation. If the patient has an area that's bruised, tender, or phlebitic, choose a vein proximal to it. Avoid flexion areas.

If your patient is elderly or has undergone repeated hospitalizations, you may have difficulty finding a suitable vein. In most cases, you should avoid veins that are hardened or sclerotic. Also try to avoid veins in the legs because circulation may be compromised more easily. If possible, avoid veins in the inner wrist and arm because they're small and thin-walled. You shouldn't use veins in the affected arm of a mastectomy patient, in an arm with an arteriovenous shunt or fistula, or in an arm that's being treated for thrombosis or cellulitis.

The size and health of the vein help determine how long the venipuncture device can remain in place before irritation develops. But the most important factor is the infusate. Drugs and solutions with high osmolarity and high or low pH will cause vein irritation sooner. Concentrated solutions of drugs and rapid infusion rates can also affect how long the I.V. site remains symptom-free.

Selecting the venipuncture device

Choosing the correct venipuncture device is as important as choosing the best available site. According to INS standards, you should select the device with the shortest length and the smallest diameter that allows for proper administration of the therapy. Selecting the device also depends on these factors:
• length of time the device will stay in place
• type of therapy
• type of procedure or surgery to be performed
• patient's activity level

• patient's age
• type of solution used (blood, for instance, will require a larger-gauge device)
• types of veins available.

Venipuncture devices. The venipuncture devices available include plastic over-the-needle catheters, through-the-needle catheters, winged infusion sets, and intermittent infusion sets. (See *Comparing venipuncture devices,* page 49.) As a rule, plastic catheters allow normal patient movement and reduce the risk of infiltration. Plus, insertion of these devices is easy. Most plastic catheters are radiopaque, which allows easy identification of catheter location.

• *Over-the-needle catheters.* The most commonly used device for peripheral I.V. therapy, an over-the-needle catheter consists of a plastic outer catheter and an inner needle that extends just beyond the catheter. The needle pulls out after insertion, leaving the catheter in place. This device's flexibility offers active patients two important advantages — greater safety and freedom of movement. Infiltration occurs less frequently than with steel-needle venipuncture devices, and armboards aren't usually necessary after insertion.

Because they have both a catheter and a needle, however, these devices are more difficult to insert than winged steel needles. So be careful to place both the inner needle and the outer catheter adequately in the vein. Typically, you should change over-the-needle catheters every 2 to 3 days. But one may stay in place longer if a patient has poor venous access and the device isn't causing any problems.

Over-the-needle peripheral vein catheters are available in lengths of

(Text continues on page 48.)

Reviewing anatomy of the skin and veins

Understanding the anatomy of the skin and veins can help you locate appropriate venipuncture sites and perform venipunctures with minimal patient discomfort.

LAYERS OF SKIN

Epidermis
• Top layer, which forms a protective covering for the dermis.
• Thickness varies in different parts of the body—usually thickest on palms of hands and soles of feet, thinnest on inner surface of limbs.
• Degree of thickness varies with age; may be thin in the elderly.

Dermis
• Highly sensitive and vascular because it contains many capillaries.
• Has thousands of nerves, which react to temperature, touch, pressure, and pain.
• Number of nerve fibers varies throughout the body; thus, certain I.V. sites are more painful than others (for example, the inner aspect of the wrist is more painful than the dorsum of the hand or the forearm).

Subcutaneous tissue
• Lies below the two layers of skin.
• Site of superficial veins.
• Loosely covers muscles and tendons, and varies in thickness.
• Potential site of cellulitis if strict aseptic technique not observed during the venipuncture and care of the I.V. site.

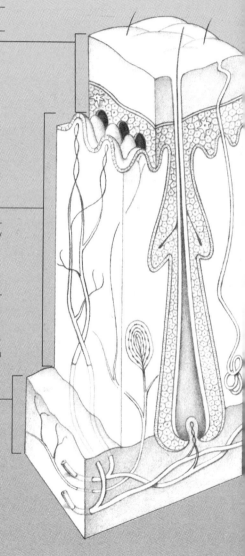

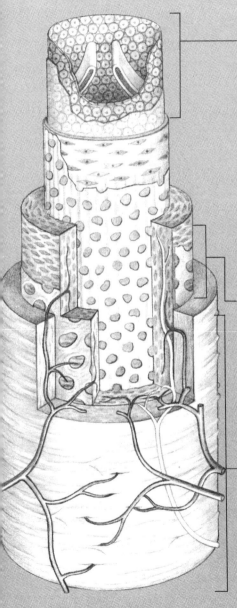

LAYERS OF THE VEINS

Tunica intima (inner layer)
• Consists of inner elastic endothelial lining, made up of layers of smooth, flat cells, which allow blood cells and platelets to flow smoothly through the blood vessels. Unnecessary movement of the venipuncture device may scratch or roughen this inner surface, causing thrombus formation.
• The valves located in this layer are in the semilunar folds of the endothelium. They're found in many veins, but especially in the veins of the limbs. Valves prevent backflow and ensure the flow of blood toward the heart.

Tunica media (middle layer)
• Consists of muscular and elastic tissue.
• Vasoconstrictor and vasodilator nerve fibers located in this layer stimulate the veins to contract and relax. They're responsible for venous spasm that can occur as a result of anxiety or of receiving I.V. fluids that are too cold.

Tunica externa (outer layer)
• Consists of connective tissue that surrounds and supports the vessel.
• Serves to hold the vessel together.

1" (2.5 cm), 1¼" (3.2 cm), and 2" (5 cm), with gauges ranging from 14 to 26. Longer-length models, used mainly in the operating room, are indicated when the insertion site is a deep vein. (See *Nurse's guide to needle and catheter gauges,* page 50.)

• *Through-the-needle catheters.* Longer plastic catheters are available for placement in long arm veins, such as the antecubital or upper arm veins. One type combines an 8" (20.3 cm) to 12" (30.5 cm) catheter with a 1½" (3.75 cm) to 2" introducer needle, which must be guarded by an enclosed shield after insertion. Patients using this device seldom require an armboard.

These longer catheters decrease the risk of infiltration, but leakage at the insertion site may occur because the needle produces a skin puncture that's larger than the catheter. These catheters are commonly used when venous access is poor or when administering caustic drugs or hypertonic solutions. They should be inserted only by skilled personnel.

• *Winged infusion sets.* You'll see two basic types of winged infusion sets — an over-the-needle catheter and a steel needle. Both have flexible wings you can grasp when inserting the device. Once the device is in place, the wings lie flat and can be taped.

The over-the-needle catheter has short, small-bore tubing between the catheter and the hub. This device is available in a ¾" length for narrow gauges and a 1" length for wider gauges. You'll find the over-the-needle catheter especially useful for hand veins.

A variation of this venipuncture device, called the Intima, has a Y-shaped design with a latex cap and can be used as an intermittent

device while an I.V. solution is infusing. Available in sizes 16G to 24G, it allows continuous and intermittent I.V. therapy with a single device, as well as simultaneous infusion of two compatible solutions.

Commonly called butterfly needles, the winged steel needles have no hub, lie flat on the skin, and make taping easy. These devices range in size from 16G to 27G and are about ¾" (1.9 cm) long. They're thin-walled and extremely sharp. Their single-needle design makes them the easiest device to insert. But because they have a steel needle instead of a plastic catheter, the risk of infiltration during patient movement is greater. Originally designed for pediatric and geriatric use, a winged steel needle should be used when a patient is in stable condition, has adequate veins, and requires I.V. fluids or medications for only a short time. It's also ideal for single I.V. push injections.

• *Intermittent infusion sets.* These devices are available as winged needle sets or as over-the-needle plastic catheters — each with an attached latex cap. However, any type of venipuncture device — plastic, steel, or long line — can be made into an intermittent device by placing a latex cap over the proximal end of the catheter. These are commonly called heparin locks because a heparin flush is instilled into the cap to keep blood from backing up into the venipuncture device and clotting. Typically, a luer-lock tip is used to prevent accidental loosening of the cap. The device should be flushed with saline solution or heparin before and after each use or at least once a day.

• *Other venipuncture devices.* The over-the-needle midline catheter (such as the Landmark catheter) absorbs plasma. After being in place

EQUIPMENT

Comparing venipuncture devices

Most I.V. infusions are delivered through three basic types of venipuncture devices: over-the-needle catheters, through-the-needle catheters, and winged infusion sets.

Over-the-needle catheter	**Through-the-needle catheter**	**Winged infusion set**
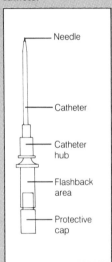	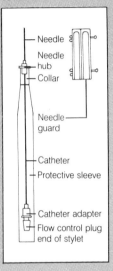	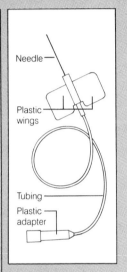

Over-the-needle catheter

Purpose: long-term therapy for the active or agitated patient
Advantages: inadvertent puncture of vein less likely than with a needle; more comfortable for the patient once it's in place; contains radiopaque thread for easy location; some units come with a syringe attached that permits easy check of blood return and prevents air from entering the vessel on insertion
Disadvantages: more difficult to insert than other devices

Through-the-needle catheter

Purpose: long-term therapy for the active or agitated patient
Advantages: inadvertent puncture of vein less likely than with a needle; more comfortable for the patient once it's in place; available in many lengths; most plastic catheters contain radiopaque thread, permitting easy location
Disadvantages: leaking at site may occur, especially in elderly patient; if needle guard not used, catheter may be severed

Winged infusion set

Purpose: short-term therapy for any cooperative adult patient; therapy of any duration for an infant or child or for an elderly patient with fragile or sclerotic veins
Advantages: easiest intravascular device to insert; ideal for I.V. push drugs
Disadvantage: may easily cause infiltration if rigid needle winged infusion device is used

Nurse's guide to needle and catheter gauges

How do you know which gauge needle and catheter to use for your patient? The answer depends on your patient's age and condition and on the type of infusion he's receiving. The following chart lists the uses and nursing considerations for the various gauges.

GAUGE	USES	NURSING CONSIDERATIONS
16	• Adolescents and adults • Major surgery • Trauma • Whenever large amounts of fluids must be infused	• Painful insertion • Requires large vein
18	• Older children, adolescents, and adults • Administration of blood and blood components and other viscous infusions	• Painful insertion • Requires large vein
20	• Children, adolescents, and adults • Suitable for most I.V. infusions	• Commonly used
22	• Infants, toddlers, children, adolescents, and adults (especially elderly) • Suitable for most I.V. infusions	• Easier to insert in small, thin, fragile veins • Slower flow rates must be maintained • More difficult to insert into tough skin
24, 26	• Neonates, infants, toddlers, school-age children, adolescents, and adults (especially elderly) • Suitable for most infusions, but flow rates are slower	• For extremely small veins—for example, small veins of fingers or veins of inner arms in elderly patients • May be difficult to insert into tough skin

for 1 hour in the antecubital space or the upper arm veins, the catheter softens and grows two gauges in diameter and 1″ in length. The over-the-needle design prevents leakage at the insertion site. Especially useful for elderly patients, this catheter allows long-term placement when venous access is limited.

Another device, the dual-lumen catheter, consists of two catheters side by side, coming together at a single tip. This device can be used to deliver two incompatible solutions. Recommended only for arm veins, the dual-lumen catheter requires greater insertion skills than other venipuncture devices because both lumens must be placed inside the vein to prevent infiltration.

Performing the venipuncture

To perform a venipuncture, you need to dilate the vein, prepare the

enipuncture site, and insert the
enipuncture device. After the
nfusion starts, you can complete
he I.V. placement by securing the
device with tape or a transparent
semipermeable dressing.

Dilating the vein

To dilate or distend a vein effectively, you need to use a tourniquet,
which traps blood in the veins by
applying enough pressure to impede
the venous flow. (See *Preparing for
venipuncture: Key steps*, page 52.)
A properly distended vein should
appear and feel round, firm, and
fully filled with blood and should
rebound when compressed. Because
the amount of trapped blood depends on the arterial circulation, a
patient who's hypotensive, very
old, or experiencing vasomotor
changes (such as septic shock) may
have inadequate filling of the peripheral blood vessels.

Before applying the tourniquet,
place the patient's arm in a dependent position to increase capillary
fill of the lower arms and hands.
If his skin is cold, warm it by rub-
bing and stroking his arm. Or cover
the entire arm with warm packs
for 5 to 10 minutes. As soon as you
remove the warm packs, apply the
tourniquet and perform the venipuncture.

Applying a tourniquet. The ideal
tourniquet can be tied easily,
doesn't roll into a thin band, stays
relatively flat, and releases easily.
Many types are available. Some
have a catch mechanism to anchor
them. Others have a wide, flat
rubber band that's secured with
Velcro. The most common type is a
soft rubber tourniquet about 2″
wide. To tie it, follow these steps.
• Place the tourniquet under the
patient's arm, about 6″ (15 cm) above

the venipuncture site. Position the arm
on the middle of the tourniquet.
• Bring the ends of the tourniquet
together, placing one on top of
the other.
• Holding one end on top of the
other, lift and stretch the tourniquet
and tuck the top tail under the
bottom tail. Don't allow the tourniquet to loosen.
• Tie the tourniquet smoothly and
snugly, being careful not to pinch
the patient's skin or pull his arm
hair.
• Leave the tourniquet in place for
no more than 2 minutes. If you can't
find a suitable vein and prepare
the venipuncture site in this amount
of time, release the tourniquet for
a few minutes. Then reapply it and
continue the procedure. You may
need to apply the tourniquet, find
the vein, remove the tourniquet,
prepare the site, and then reapply
the tourniquet for the venipuncture.

Keep the tourniquet as flat as
possible. It should be snug but not
uncomfortably tight. If it's too tight,
it'll impede arterial as well as venous blood flow. Check the patient's
radial pulse. If you can't feel it,
the tourniquet is too tight and must
be loosened. Also loosen and reapply the tourniquet if the patient
complains of severe tightness.

Once you've applied the tourniquet, distend the vein by following
these steps.
• Have the patient open and close
his fist tightly four to six times.
• Flick the skin over the vein with
one or two sharp snaps of your
forefinger. This is less traumatic
than slapping the skin, yet it
achieves the same effect of distend-
ing the vein.
• Rub or stroke the skin upward
toward the tourniquet.
• If the vein still feels small and
unfirm, release the tourniquet.

Preparing for venipuncture: Key steps

These illustrations show key steps you'll perform when dilating the patient's vein or cleaning the venipuncture site.

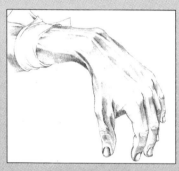

Dilating the patient's vein
Apply the tourniquet close to the venipuncture site you've chosen—for example, on the mid-forearm for hand veins. After the tourniquet is applied, the vein should look and feel rounded and swollen with blood, and the skin below the tourniquet should appear darker from trapped blood.

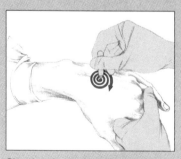

Cleaning the venipuncture site
After you've dilated the vein, clean the venipuncture site, starting at the center and wiping outward with a circular motion. Make sure you're wearing gloves for this step.

Reapply it a little tighter and closer to the venipuncture site than before.
• If the vein still isn't well distended, remove the tourniquet, apply a warm pack for 5 minutes and reapply the tourniquet. This is especially helpful if the patient's skin feels cool.

A tourniquet that's applied too tightly or kept in place too long may cause increased bruising—especially in elderly patients whose veins are fragile. Release the tourniquet as soon as you've placed the venipuncture device into the vein. You'll know the device is in the vein when you see blood in the venipuncture device's flashback chamber.

Preparing the venipuncture site

Before performing the venipuncture, you may need to administer a local anesthetic, and you'll need to clean the site and stabilize the vein. Stabilizing the vein helps ensure a successful venipuncture the first time and decreases the chances of bruising the vein. Bruising occurs when the tip of the venipuncture device repeatedly probes a moving vein wall, nicking the vein and causing it to leak blood. When such damage occurs, the vein can't be reused immediately. So a new venipuncture site must be found, and the patient must experience the discomfort of another needle puncture.

Cleaning the venipuncture site.
Place an absorbent pad under the venipuncture site. Then put on gloves. Clip the hair over the insertion site. Next, clean the skin with a thin coat of a solution such as povidone-iodine, tincture of iodine, or 70% alcohol. Wipe the skin, starting at the center of the insertion site and moving outward with a circular motion. To reduce the risk

f contamination, use a swab stick or swab ampule rather than a cleansing pad. Be careful not to go over an area you've already cleaned. Allow the solution to dry thoroughly (this takes about 30 to 60 seconds).

Using a local anesthetic. Many doctors order a local anesthetic before venipuncture, although the practice isn't endorsed by the INS. If you'll be administering a local anesthetic, check the patient's record for an allergy to lidocaine or iodine. Also, ask him if he's allergic to any drugs or other substances — particularly these two. Then describe the procedure to him and explain that it'll reduce the pain of the venipuncture.

Now administer the local anesthetic, as ordered. You'll administer only a small amount, and the anesthetic will work in 2 to 3 seconds. Lidocaine numbs pain but allows the patient to feel touch and pressure. (See *Administering a local anesthetic,* page 54.)

Stabilizing the vein. Next, stabilize the vein by stretching the skin and holding it taut. Lightly press it with your fingertips about 1½" from the intended insertion site. The vein should feel round, firm, fully engorged, and resilient. Remove your fingertips. If the vein returns to its original position and appears larger than it did before you applied the tourniquet, the vein is adequately distended. (See *How to stabilize veins,* page 55.)

To help prevent the veins from rolling, lift the tied tourniquet from the skin and pull the skin toward the shoulder. Then lower the tied tourniquet. This will help secure the veins, particularly in elderly patients with loose skin and loosely anchored veins.

Insertion

Once you've prepared the venipuncture site, you're ready to insert the venipuncture device. The first step is to position the device correctly. Then, insert it into the vein, using either the direct or the indirect approach. Finally, advance the device fully into the vein, either before or during infusion. If ordered, collect a blood sample when you perform the venipuncture.

Positioning the venipuncture device. While still wearing gloves, grasp the device, using the appropriate method:

1. • *Over-the-needle catheter.* Grasp the plastic hub with your dominant hand, remove the cover, and examine the device. If the edge isn't smooth, discard and replace the device. (See *Inserting an over-the-needle catheter,* page 56.)

2. • *Through-the-needle catheter.* Grasp the needle hub with one hand and unsnap the needle cover. With the skin taut and anchored, position the device with the bevel up and the flashback chamber visible. Firmly hold this chamber, being careful not to touch the catheter.

3. • *Winged infusion set.* Hold the edges of the wings between your thumb and forefinger, with the bevel facing upward. Then squeeze the wings together.

Inserting the venipuncture device. Tell the patient that you're about to insert the device. To use the direct approach, place the bevel up and enter the skin directly over the vein at a 30- to 45-degree angle (deeper veins require a wider angle). To use the indirect approach, enter the skin slightly adjacent to the vein, then direct the needle into the side of the vein wall. This approach reduces the risk of perforating the

Administering a local anesthetic

Many doctors order a local anesthetic when starting peripheral I.V. therapy, although the Intravenous Nurses Society (INS) doesn't recommend the practice. If you'll be administering a local anesthetic, use the following procedure:

• Using a U-100 insulin syringe with a 27G needle, draw up 0.1 ml of lidocaine 1% without epinephrine.
• Clean the venipuncture site.
• Insert the needle next to the vein, introducing about one-third of it into the skin subcutaneously at a 30-degree angle (as shown). The side approach carries less risk of accidental vein puncture (indicated by blood appearing in the syringe). If the vein is deep, however, inject the lidocaine over the top of it. Just be careful not to inject lidocaine into the vein.

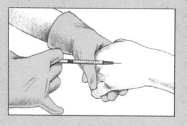

• Hold your thumb on the plunger of the syringe during insertion to avoid unnecessary movement once the needle is under the skin.
• Without aspirating, quickly inject the lidocaine until a small wheal appears (as shown). You may not have to administer the entire amount in the syringe.

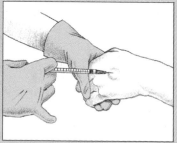

• Quickly withdraw the syringe and massage the wheal with an alcohol swab. This will make the wheal disappear so the vein won't be hidden. However, you'll see a small pinprick of blood. The skin numbness will last about 30 minutes.
• Insert the venipuncture device into the vein.

back vein wall. If the vein is bifurcated (looks like an inverted V), penetrate the skin about ½" (1.25 cm) in front of the bifurcation and proceed into the vein lumen.

Insert the device with a steady, smooth motion while keeping the skin taut. Usually you'll know the device is in the vein when you meet resistance during insertion and when you see blood return in the flashback chamber. (You may not see blood return with a small vein.) Don't expect to always feel a "pop," or a sense of release, when the device enters the vein. This usually

occurs only when a larger gauge venipuncture device (20G or larger) enters a large, thick-walled vein. It also tends to occur more often with young patients.

Advancing the venipuncture device.
As soon as the device enters the vein, lower it until it's almost parallel with the skin. This lifts the tip so it doesn't penetrate the back wall of the vein. Then, if you're using an over-the-needle catheter, advance the device to at least half of its length. After blood return is evident, you'll advance the catheter

ow to stabilize veins

To help ensure successful venipuncture, you need to stabilize your patient's vein by stretching the skin and holding it taut. The stretching technique you'll use varies with different venipuncture sites.

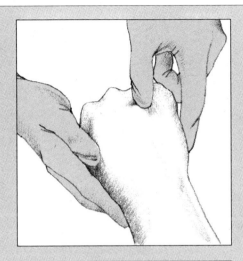

VEIN	STRETCHING TECHNIQUE
Hand veins	Stretch the patient's hand and wrist downward and hold your thumb as shown.
Cephalic vein above wrist	Have the patient make a tight fist. Then stretch his fist laterally downward and immobilize the skin with the thumb of your other hand.
Basilic vein at outer arm	Have the patient make a tight fist and flex his elbow. While standing behind the flexed arm, retract the skin away from the site and anchor the vein with your thumb. As an alternative, rotate the patient's extended lower arm inward and approach the vein from behind the arm. (This position may be difficult for the patient to maintain.)
Inner aspect of wrist	Extend the patient's open hand backward from the wrist. Anchor the vein with your thumb below the insertion site.
Inner arm	Extend the patient's closed fist backward from the wrist. Anchor the vein with your thumb above the wrist.
Antecubital fossa	Have the patient form a tight fist and extend his arm completely. Anchor the skin with your thumb, about 2″ to 3″ (5 to 7.5 cm) below the antecubital fossa.
Saphenous vein of ankle	Extend the patient's foot downward and inward. Anchor the vein with your thumb, about 2″ to 3″ below the ankle.
Dorsum of foot	Pull the patient's foot downward. Anchor the vein with your thumb, about 2″ to 3″ below the vein (usually near the toes).

Inserting an over-the-needle catheter

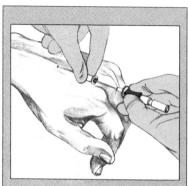

Insert the device through the skin and into the vein. Then lower the device until it's almost parallel to the skin. Advance the device to at least half its length, when you should see blood in the flashback chamber. If you're advancing the catheter before starting the infusion, leave the needle in place. Then advance the catheter to its hub and withdraw the needle, as shown.

completely, either while infusing I.V. solution or before.

To advance the catheter while infusing I.V. solution, release the tourniquet and remove the inner needle. Using aseptic technique, attach the I.V. tubing and begin the infusion. While stabilizing the vein with one hand, use the other to advance the catheter into the vein. When the catheter is advanced, slow the I.V. flow rate. This method reduces the risk of puncturing the back vein wall because the catheter is advanced without the steel needle and because the rapid flow dilates the vein.

To advance the catheter before starting the infusion, first release the tourniquet. While stabilizing the vein with one hand, use the other

to advance the catheter up to the hub. Next, remove the inner needle and, using aseptic technique, quickly attach the I.V. tubing. This method often results in less blood being spilled.

When using a winged infusion set advance the needle fully if possible and hold it in place. Release the tourniquet, open the administration set clamp slightly, and check for free flow or infiltration. Then tape the infusion set in place, using the chevron method to prevent needle movement, which could cause irritation and phlebitis.

After the venipuncture device has been inserted, clean the skin completely before you remove your gloves and wash your hands. If necessary, dispose of the inner needle in a needle receptacle. Then regulate the flow rate.

Inserting an intermittent infusion device. If your patient requires intermittent infusion of solutions or medications, you'll need to insert an intermittent infusion device. Also called a heparin lock, this device consists of a winged steel needle with tubing or a catheter that ends in a resealable rubber injection port. Once it's filled with dilute heparin or saline solution to prevent blood clot formation, the device maintains venous access in patients who must receive I.V. medications regularly or intermittently but who don't require continuous infusion of fluids. Unlike a keep-vein-open line, it minimizes the risk of fluid overload and electrolyte imbalance. It's also less expensive and reduces the risk of contamination by eliminating the continuous use of I.V. solution containers and administration sets. The device increases patient comfort and mobility, reduces patient anxiety, and allows you to collect blood

amples without repeated venipunctures. If your patient has a clotting
disorder or uncontrolled bleeding,
use 1 to 2 ml of sterile normal
saline solution instead of heparin.

Insert a heparin lock as you'd
insert any other venipuncture device, with these exceptions:

• After removing the set from its
package, wipe the port with an
alcohol swab and inject a dilute heparin or saline solution to fill the
tubing and needle. This removes air
from the system, preventing air
embolus formation.

• After performing the venipuncture, tape the set in place, using the
chevron method or an accepted
alternative. Loop the tubing so that
the injection port is easily accessible. In some hospitals, nurses use an
elastic net dressing over the top of
the heparin lock and sterile dressing, leaving the port exposed.

• After applying a sterile dressing,
again flush the set with heparin
or saline solution to prevent clot formation.

• In the nurses' notes, record the
date and time of insertion and the
type and gauge of the needle.

Regularly flush the heparin lock to
maintain patency. Follow hospital
policy regarding the type of solution
and frequency of flushing.

If the patient feels a burning
sensation as you inject the heparin
or saline solution, stop the injection
and check the catheter or needle
placement. If it's in the vein, inject
the heparin or saline solution at a
lower rate to minimize irritation.

If the doctor orders an I.V. infusion discontinued and a heparin lock
inserted in its place, you can convert the existing line into a heparin
lock. Most venipuncture devices
can be converted by disconnecting
the I.V. tubing and inserting a male
adapter plug into the device. (See

*Converting an I.V. line into a hepa-
rin lock,* page 58.)

Insertion in deeper veins. Sometimes, when a superficial vein isn't
available, you'll have to insert the
venipuncture device into a deep
vein. If the deep vein isn't visible,
palpate the area with your fingertips
until you feel it. Clean the skin
over the vein with an alcohol swab;
the moisture helps highlight the
vein, making it appear as a faint
shadow under the skin. Aim the device directly over the outlined vein.
Stretch the skin with your fingertips, while inserting the venipuncture device about 1½" distal to your
fingertips. Insert one-half or two-
thirds of its length to be sure that
both the needle and catheter are
in the vein lumen. When you see
blood in the flashback chamber,
remove the inner steel needle and
advance the catheter with or without infusing fluid.

Collecting a blood sample. If ordered, collect a blood sample while
performing the venipuncture. First,
gather the equipment you'll need:
one or more evacuated tubes, a 19G
needle, an appropriate-size syringe
without a needle, and a protective
pad. Then follow these steps:

• When the venipuncture device is
correctly placed, remove the inner
needle if you're using an over-
the-needle device.

• Leaving the tourniquet tied, place
the pad underneath the site to
protect the bed linen.

• Attach the syringe to the venipuncture device's hub and withdraw
the appropriate amount of blood.

• Release the tourniquet and disconnect the syringe.

• Attach the I.V. tubing, regulate
the flow rate, and stabilize the
device.

Converting an I.V. line into a heparin lock

Two types of male adapter plugs allow you to convert an existing I.V. line into a heparin lock for intermittent infusion of medication. To make the conversion:
• prime the male adapter plug with dilute heparin or saline solution
• clamp the I.V. tubing and remove the administration set from the catheter or needle hub
• insert the male adapter plug (see illustrations)
• inject the remaining dilute heparin or saline solution to fill the line and to prevent clot formation.

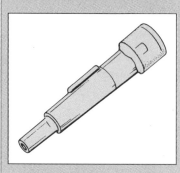

This long male adapter plug slides into place.

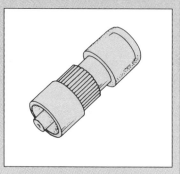

This short male luer-lock adapter plug twists into place.

• Attach the 19G needle to the syringe and insert the blood into th evacuated tubes.
• Remove the needle and syringe and dispose of them properly. Then complete the I.V. line placement.

Securing the venipuncture device

After the infusion begins, you need to secure the venipuncture device a the insertion site. You can do this using tape or a transparent semipe meable dressing. After applying tape or the dressing, be sure to labe it with the date and time of the insertion, the type and gauge of the venipuncture device, and the initial of the person inserting it.

If the arm or leg must be immobi lized during infusion, you may need to apply an armboard. Remem ber to document your interventions carefully after you've performed the venipuncture.

Taping at the I.V. site. If hospital policy requires, place a small amount of antiseptic ointment directly over the insertion site. (This ointment should be applied daily.) Apply an adhesive bandage or a sterile 2″ × 2″ gauze pad directly over the insertion site. Then apply 1″ (2.5 cm) piece of tape over the sterile dressing, being careful not t tape over the edge of the venipuncture device's hub. Using the chevro method, wrap a ½″ (1.25 cm) piece of tape at the hub to stabilize the device. Apply another piece of tape over the chevron tape to keep the hub from moving. Then loop the tubing and tape it. (See *Taping techniques.*)

Use as little tape as possible and don't let the tape ends meet. This reduces the risk of a tourniquet effect should infiltration occur. If necessary, remove excess hair from

aping techniques

If you'll be using tape to secure the venipuncture device to the insertion site, use one of the four basic methods described below.

CHEVRON METHOD

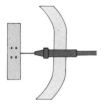 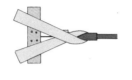 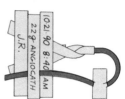

1. Cover the venipuncture site with an adhesive strip or a 2″ × 2″ sterile gauze pad. Then cut a long strip of ½″ (1.25-cm) tape. Place it, sticky side up, under the needle, parallel to the short strip of tape.

2. Cross the ends of the tape over the needle so that the tape sticks to the patient's skin.

3. Apply a piece of 1″ (2.5-cm) tape across the two wings of the chevron. Loop the tubing and secure it with another piece of 1″ tape. On the tape, write the date and time of insertion, the type and gauge of the needle, and your initials.

U METHOD

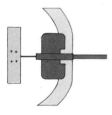 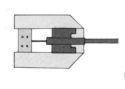 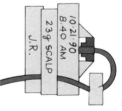

1. Cover the venipuncture site with an adhesive strip or a 2″ × 2″ sterile gauze pad. Then cut a strip of ½″ tape. With the sticky side up, place it under the tubing.

2. Bring each side of the tape up, folding it over the wings of the needle, as shown here. Press it down, parallel to the tubing.

3. Now apply tape as you would with the chevron method. On the tape, write the date and time of insertion, the type and gauge of the needle or catheter, and your initials.

(continued)

Taping techniques *(continued)*

TWO-TAPE METHOD

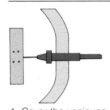 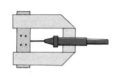 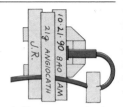

1. Cover the venipuncture site with an adhesive strip or a 2″ × 2″ sterile gauze pad. Then place a 2″ (5-cm) strip of ½″ tape, sticky side up, under the needle.

2. Fold the tape ends over and affix them to the patient's skin in a U shape, as shown here.

3. Place a second strip of ½″ tape, sticky side down, over the needle hub. On the tape, write the date and time of insertion, the type and gauge of the needle or catheter, and your initials.

With this method, you can remove the upper strip of tape to check the insertion site while the lower strip anchors the needle.

H METHOD

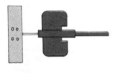 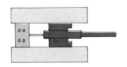 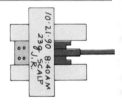

1. Cover the venipuncture site with an adhesive strip or a 2″ × 2″ gauze pad. Then cut three strips of 1″ tape.

2. Place one strip of tape over each wing, keeping the tape parallel to the needle.

3. Now place the other strip of tape perpendicular to the first two. Put it either directly on top of the wings or just below the wings, directly on top of the tubing. On the last piece of tape, write the date and time of insertion, the type and gauge of the needle or catheter, and your initials.

he site before you apply the tape. Removing hair improves visibility of he veins and the site and reduces pain when the tape is removed. Don't allow the tape to cover the patient's skin beyond the device's ip. This could obscure swelling and redness. If the patient has had a previous allergic reaction to tape, use a nonallergenic tape — preferably one that's lightweight and easy to remove. Usually, paper tape isn't satisfactory for I.V. sites because it shreds and is difficult to remove.

Depending on your hospital's policy, remove the old dressing every 1 to 2 days and clean the insertion site with povidone-iodine. As always, start at the center and wipe outward, using a circular motion. If residue remains on the skin, clean it with alcohol. Allow the skin to dry, then apply tape.

Applying a transparent dressing. To prevent infection, nurses in many hospitals now use a transparent semipermeable dressing on the insertion site instead of tape. (See *How to apply a transparent semipermeable dressing.*) This dressing allows air to pass through it, but it's impervious to microorganisms. If he dressing remains intact, daily changes aren't necessary. Other advantages include fewer skin reactions and a clearly visible insertion site (especially helpful in detecting the early signs of phlebitis and swelling). Because the tape is waterproof, it protects the site from contamination should it become wet. And because the dressing adheres well to the skin, there's less chance of accidentally dislodging the venipuncture device.

Using a stretch net. A way to make he venipuncture device more secure is to apply a stretch net to the

How to apply a transparent semipermeable dressing

Instead of using tape to secure the I.V. insertion site, you can apply a transparent semipermeable dressing. Here's how:

● Make sure the insertion site is clean and dry.
● Remove the dressing from the package and, using aseptic technique, remove the protective seal. Avoid touching the sterile surface.
● Place the dressing directly over the insertion site and the hub, as shown. Don't cover the tubing. Also, don't stretch the dressing; doing so may cause itching.
● Tuck the dressing around and under the catheter hub to make the site occlusive to microorganisms.

To remove the dressing, grasp one corner, then lift and stretch.

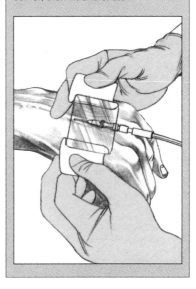

affected limb. (If you'll be using the net on the patient's hand, you'll need to cut a hole in the net sleeve for his thumb.) The net reduces the risk of accidental dislodgment, especially among patients who are confused or very active.

Using an armboard. An armboard helps prevent unnecessary motion that could cause infiltration or inflammation. This device is sometimes necessary when a venipuncture device is inserted near a joint or in the dorsum of the hand, or it may be used along with a restraint for confused or disoriented patients. Because armboards don't prevent rotation, however, they can't always prevent infiltration. Proper placement of the tip of the device away from a flexion area usually avoids the need for an armboard.

To determine if your patient needs an armboard, move his arm through its full range of motion while watching the I.V. flow rate. If the rate stops during movement, you'll need to use an armboard. Choose one that's long enough to prevent flexion and extension at the tip of the device. You should cover the board with a soft material and apply it with tape that's padded with folded gauze or paper tissue. Leave the area of the device's tip uncovered by tape so you can see it.

Remove the armboard periodically to decrease the risk of complications. An armboard applied too tightly could cause nerve and tendon damage. If you need to apply a restraint, apply it to the armboard, not to the patient's arm.

Documenting the venipuncture
When you start an I.V. line, be sure to document the following:
• the date and time of the venipuncture
• the number of the solution container (if required by hospital policy)
• the type and amount of solution

• the name and dosage of additives in the solution
• the type of venipuncture device used, including the length and gauge
• the venipuncture site
• the number of insertion attempts if more than one
• the flow rate
• any adverse reactions and the actions taken to correct them
• patient teaching and evidence of patient understanding
• the name of the person initiating the infusion.

Maintaining peripheral I.V. therapy

After the I.V. infusion starts, you'll need to focus on maintaining therapy and preventing complications. This involves routine care measures such as regular dressing and tubing changes. Plus, it involves special care measures, such as administering additive infusions. You also must be able to meet the special needs of pediatric, elderly, or home care patients who require I.V. therapy. Finally, you'll need to discontinue the infusion.

Routine care
Routine care during I.V. therapy includes regularly changing the tubing and dressings, the solution, and the administration set as well as rotating I.V. sites. These measures help prevent complications. Routine care measures also give you an opportunity to observe the I.V. site for signs of inflammation or infection—two of the most common complications.

You should perform all routine

care procedures according to your hospital's policy. Remember to wash your hands before any procedure and to wear gloves whenever performing a procedure that requires you to work near the venipuncture site.

Dressing changes. You'll change the I.V. dressings using aseptic technique every 24 to 48 hours and whenever the dressings become soiled, wet, or loose. Before performing a dressing change, gather this equipment: povidone-iodine or alcohol swab; povidone-iodine ointment or another antimicrobial ointment (if your hospital policy requires it); adhesive bandage, sterile 2″ × 2″ gauze pad, or transparent semipermeable dressing; 1″ adhesive tape; and sterile gloves.

To change a dressing, follow these steps:
• Wash your hands and put on the sterile gloves.
• Hold the needle or catheter in place with your nondominant hand to prevent accidental movement or dislodgment, which could lead to infiltration. Then gently remove the tape and the dressing.
• Assess the venipuncture site for signs of infection (redness and tenderness); infiltration (coolness, blanching, and edema); and thrombophlebitis (redness, firmness, pain along the path of the vein, and edema). If you detect these signs, apply pressure to the area with a sterile 2″ × 2″ gauze pad and remove the catheter or needle. Maintain pressure on the area until the bleeding stops, and apply an adhesive bandage. Then, using new equipment, start the I.V. infusion at another site. If you don't detect complications, hold the needle or catheter at the hub and carefully clean around the site with the povi-

done-iodine or alcohol swab. Work from the site outward to avoid introducing pathogens into the cleaned area. Allow the area to dry completely.
• If hospital policy requires, apply povidone-iodine ointment or another antimicrobial ointment. Then cover the site with the adhesive bandage or the gauze pad and retape the site, or apply the transparent semipermeable dressing.

Changing the I.V. solution. To avoid microbial growth, you shouldn't allow any I.V. container to hang for more than 24 hours. Before changing the I.V. container, you'll need to obtain a new container. Remember to check the new container for cracks, leaks, and other damage. Also check the solution for discoloration, turbidity, and particulates. Note the date and time the solution was mixed and the expiration date.

Then follow these steps:
• Wash your hands.
• Clamp the line, remove the spike from the old container, and quickly insert the spike into the new one.
• Hang the new container and adjust the flow rate.

Changing the administration set. Change the administration set according to your hospital's policy (usually every 48 hours) and whenever you note or suspect contamination. If possible, try to change the administration set when you hang a new solution container. Before changing a set, gather this equipment: an I.V. administration set, a sterile 2″ × 2″ gauze pad, adhesive tape for labeling, hemostats (optional), and sterile gloves.
• Wash your hands and put on the gloves.
• Reduce the I.V. flow rate. Then remove the old spike from the con-

tainer and place the cover of the new spike over it loosely.
• Keeping the old spike upright and above the patient's heart level, insert the new spike into the I.V. container and prime the system.
• Place the sterile gauze pad under the needle or hub of the plastic catheter to create a sterile field.
• Disconnect the old tubing from the venipuncture device, being careful not to dislodge or move the I.V. device. If you have trouble disconnecting the old tubing, use a pair of hemostats to hold the hub securely while twisting and removing the end of the tubing. Or use one pair of hemostats on the venipuncture device and another pair on the hard plastic of the luer-lock end of the administration set. Then pull the hemostats in opposite directions.
Note: Don't clamp the hemostats shut; this may crack the tubing adapter or the venipuncture device.
• Using aseptic technique, quickly attach the new primed tubing to the I.V. device.
• Adjust the flow to the prescribed rate.
• Label the new tubing with the date and time of the tubing change.

Changing the I.V. site. Rotate the I.V. site every 48 to 72 hours, if possible. Sometimes, limited venous access will prevent you from changing sites this frequently. In this case, be sure to inspect the site frequently and to change it if you note redness, pain, or swelling. Be prepared to change the entire system, including the venipuncture device, if you detect signs of thrombophlebitis, cellulitis, or I.V. therapy-related bacteremia.

Documentation. Record dressing, tubing, and solution changes, and note the condition of the venipunc-

ture site. If you obtain a specimen for culture and sensitivity testing, record the date and time and the name of the doctor.

Special care procedures

Many of your responsibilities in maintaining peripheral I.V. therapy are routine, but you must also be prepared to handle special situations. For instance, you need to know how to administer additive infusions. Also, when venipuncture isn't possible, you may need to assist with venesection or use hypodermoclysis.

Additive infusions. To infuse two compatible solutions simultaneously, connect an administration set with an attached 20G 1″ needle to the secondary solution container and prime the tubing. Hang the container at the same level as the primary solution. Then clean a Y-site in the lower part of the primary tubing, using a povidone-iodine or alcohol swab. Attach your secondary infusion set to the Y-site. Adjust each infusion rate independently. With this setup, you don't have a backcheck valve above the Y-site, so one solution may flow back into the other.

To piggyback an I.V. drug into a primary line, you should use an add-a-line administration set.

Venesection and hypodermoclysis.
Though these procedures are seldom performed anymore, you should be familiar with them. Each provides a way of entering a peripheral vein when you can't use the usual venipuncture techniques because of obesity, venous collapse or sclerosis, or vasoconstriction from massive, rapid blood loss. The procedures are also performed on patients whose usable veins are exhausted.

In venesection, also called venous cutdown, the doctor makes a small incision in the skin over the vein. He divides subcutaneous tissues, isolates the vein, and temporarily ties a ligature around it. Then he makes a small incision in the vein, inserts a 3″ to 6″ plastic catheter into it, and anchors the catheter with a suture. The catheter can remain in place for several days.

In hypodermoclysis, you use the subcutaneous route to achieve absorption of I.V. isotonic hydration fluids. This procedure is still performed in some long-term care facilities and at home. Usually reserved for infants and elderly patients, hypodermoclysis can't be used for patients suffering from shock or severe electrolyte imbalance because the I.V. solution must be iso-osmolar or tissue irritation will develop.

Patients with special needs

Pediatric and elderly patients receiving I.V. therapy pose special nursing challenges. So do patients who are scheduled to continue receiving I.V. therapy at home. For pediatric and elderly patients, you need to understand how age-related differences in the skin and veins affect I.V. line insertion and maintenance. For home care patients, you need to provide thorough patient teaching about routine procedures and emergency care.

Pediatric patients. Inserting a venipuncture device in an infant or toddler can prove difficult because his veins are imbedded in fat and hard to isolate. Usually, you'll find that performing a venipuncture on a premature infant is easier. That's because he has less fat, making his veins more prominent.

• *I.V. insertion sites.* In infants, the

Identifying scalp veins

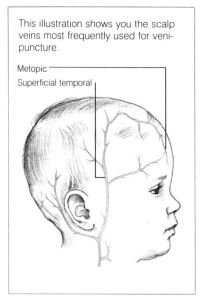

This illustration shows you the scalp veins most frequently used for venipuncture.

Metopic
Superficial temporal

best sites for I.V. insertion include the hands, feet, antecubital fossa, inner wrist, and especially the scalp, which has an abundant supply of veins. (See *Identifying scalp veins.*) The head veins most frequently used are the bilateral superficial temporal veins above the ear and the metopic vein running down the middle of the forehead. Scalp veins are extremely fragile and should be used only on infants under age 6 months; an older child is more likely to move his head and dislodge the venipuncture device. In toddlers, dorsal foot veins can be used, but dorsal hand veins allow the greatest mobility.

• *Venipuncture techniques.* Before performing a venipuncture on a scalp vein, palpate to ensure you have a vein—not an artery. In the scalp, arteries and veins may look similar. But you'll feel a pulse with an artery, not with a vein.

Consider using a topical anesthetic to decrease discomfort. And use clove-hitch and mummy restraints as necessary. Don't use a tourniquet for scalp vein venipuncture; if you need a tourniquet effect, tie a rubber band around the scalp well above the eyes and ears. Insert the venipuncture device caudally to make taping easier. When you see a blood return (usually it'll be slight), remove the rubber band.

No matter which vein you're using, a small-diameter winged over-the-needle catheter (commonly called a scalp vein needle) is preferred for infants and young children. This device is less likely to injure the vein. Over-the-needle catheters are also recommended for long-term therapy, total parenteral nutrition, and antibiotic therapy when venous access is poor.

You'll find that stabilizing the I.V. site can be difficult in pediatric patients. Tape the site as you would for an adult — so the skin over the tip of the venipuncture device is easily visible. Avoid overtaping the I.V. site; doing so makes it harder to inspect the site and surrounding tissues. Instead, cover the site with a stretch net, which can be rolled back easily for inspection. Some clinicians tape a plastic medicine cup over the insertion site to protect it.

• *Intraosseous infusion.* You should also be familiar with a recently revived emergency procedure — intraosseous infusion, which has been replacing emergency venesections. In this procedure, used for children under age 3, a bone marrow needle is placed in the medullary cavity of bones, usually in the distal end of the femur or the proximal or distal ends of the tibia. The I.V. solution is then infused directly into the bone marrow, which is rich in blood. Usually performed by emergency personnel, this procedure is indicated to provide resuscitative fluids medication, and blood until a vein can be used for I.V. administration.

Elderly patients. Because an elderly person's veins are usually more prominent and his skin less resistant, you'll find venipuncture easier than with pediatric patients. However, the normal aging process also presents certain drawbacks. Because the tissues become looser, you'll have more difficulty stabilizing the vein. And because veins become more fragile, you'll need to perform the venipuncture quickly and efficiently to avoid excessive bruising. You'll also need to remove the tourniquet promptly to prevent increased vascular pressure from bleeding through the vein wall around the insertion site.

Typically, an elderly person's veins appear blue and tortuous because of the skin's increased transparency and decreased elasticity. They'll also appear large if venous pressure is adequate. Winged steel needles are commonly used as I.V. insertion devices for elderly patient because they are less thrombogenic can be easily manipulated, and lie flat against the skin to provide a stable site for the device. But be aware that these needles increase the risk of infiltration.

To help stabilize the vein for insertion, stretch the skin proximal to the insertion site and anchor it with a tourniquet. Or you can place the arm in a dependent position; the veins won't be as firm and stable with this method, but it reduces the amount of vein bruising. Usually, smaller, shorter venipuncture devices work best with elderly patients' fragile veins.

Home care patients. Most patients receiving I.V. therapy at home will have a central venous line. But if you care for a patient who will be going home with a peripheral line, you should teach him to care for the I.V. site and identify certain complications. If he must observe movement restrictions, make sure he understands them.

Teach the patient how to examine the site and tell him to notify his doctor if he detects redness, swelling, or discomfort; a moist dressing; or blood in the tubing. Also, tell the patient to report any problems with the I.V. line — for instance, if the solution stops infusing or if an alarm goes off on the infusion pump or controller. Explain that the I.V. site must be changed at established intervals by a home care nurse, and work out a tentative schedule with him.

If the patient is using an intermittent infusion device, such as a heparin lock, teach him how and when to flush it. Finally, teach him to document daily whether the I.V. site is free of pain, swelling, and redness.

Complications of therapy

The potential complications of therapy include infection, phlebitis, circulatory overload, and allergic reactions. Complications may be associated with the venipuncture, the infusion, or the medication being administered. They may be local or systemic, or they may begin locally and become systemic — for instance, when an infection at the venipuncture site progresses to septicemia. Fortunately, you can minimize or prevent most complications by using proper insertion techniques and carefully monitoring the patient.

Extravasation. Perhaps the greatest threat to a patient receiving I.V. therapy is extravasation — the leakage of infusing fluid from a vein into the surrounding tissues. Also called infiltration, extravasation occurs when the venipuncture device punctures or slips out of the vein wall. The risk of extravasation may be as much as 70% greater with a steel needle than with a plastic catheter, depending on the skill of the person performing the venipuncture.

Extravasation involving steel needles can occur any time after you start an infusion. If a plastic catheter is used, extravasation is more likely to occur one or more days after insertion — usually as a result of the flexible catheter tip penetrating the vein wall during the infusion.

With either venipuncture device, the risk of extravasation increases whenever you insert it near a joint. Extravasation also occurs when the tip of the venipuncture device isn't inserted far enough. In this case, part of the tip lies outside the vein, and extravasation quickly develops.

The type of fluid being infused determines how much discomfort the patient feels during extravasation. Isotonic fluids usually don't cause much discomfort. Fluids with an acidic or alkaline pH, or those that are more than slightly hypertonic, are usually more irritating. But don't depend on the patient to complain of discomfort from extravasation. Large amounts of I.V. fluid — as much as a liter, in fact — can escape into the surrounding tissues without the patient knowing it. (See *Risks of peripheral I.V. therapy,* pages 68 to 72.)

If complications occur, document the signs and symptoms, patient complaints, name of the doctor

(*Text continues on page 72.*)

COMPLICATIONS

Risks of peripheral I.V. therapy

As with any invasive vascular procedure, peripheral I.V. therapy carries associated risks. Complications may be local, such as phlebitis, or systemic, such as circulatory overload or infection. This chart lists some common complications along with their signs and symptoms, possible causes, and nursing interventions, including preventive measures.

SIGNS AND SYMPTOMS	POSSIBLE CAUSES	NURSING INTERVENTIONS
Local complications		
Phlebitis		
• Tenderness at tip of venipuncture device and above	• Poor blood flow around venipuncture device	• Remove venipuncture device.
• Redness at tip of catheter and along vein	• Friction from catheter movement in vein	• Apply warm pack.
• Puffy area over vein	• Venipuncture device left in vein too long	• Notify doctor if patient has fever.
• Vein hard on palpation	• Clotting at catheter tip (thrombophlebitis)	• Document patient's condition and your interventions.
• Elevated temperature	• Solution with high or low pH or high osmolarity	*Prevention:*
		• Restart infusion using larger vein for irritating infusate, or restart with smaller-gauge device to ensure adequate blood flow.
		• Use filter to reduce risk of phlebitis.
		• Tape venipuncture device securely to prevent motion.
Extravasation		
• Swelling at and above I.V. site (may extend along entire limb)	• Venipuncture device dislodged from vein or perforated vein	• Remove venipuncture device.
• Discomfort, burning, or pain at site		• Apply ice (early) or warm soaks (later) to aid absorption.
• Feeling of tightness at site		• Elevate limb.
• Decreased skin temperature around site		• Check for pulse and capillary refill periodically to assess circulation.
• Blanching at site		• Restart infusion above infiltration site or in another limb.
• Continuing fluid infusion even when vein is occluded, although rate may decrease		• Document patient's condition and your interventions.
• Absent backflow of blood		*Prevention:*
• Slower flow rate		• Check I.V. site frequently (especially when using I.V. pump).
		• Don't obscure area above site with tape.
		• Teach patient to observe I.V. site and report pain or swelling.
Catheter dislodgment		
• Loose tape	• Loosened tape or tubing snagged in bedclothes, resulting in partial retraction of catheter	• If no infiltration occurs, retape without pushing catheter back into vein.
• Catheter partly backed out of vein		*Prevention:*
• Infusate infiltrating		• Tape venipuncture device securely on insertion.

COMPLICATIONS

Risks of peripheral I.V. therapy *(continued)*

SIGNS AND SYMPTOMS	POSSIBLE CAUSES	NURSING INTERVENTIONS
Local complications *(continued)*		
Occlusion • No increase in flow rate when I.V. container is raised • Blood backup in line • Discomfort at insertion site	• I.V. flow interrupted • Heparin lock not flushed • Blood backup in line when patient walks • Hypercoagulable patient • Line clamped too long	• Use mild flush injection. Don't force injection. If unsuccessful, reinsert I.V. line. *Prevention:* • Maintain I.V. flow rate. • Flush promptly after intermittent piggyback administration. • Have patient walk with his arm folded to chest to reduce risk of blood backup.
Vein irritation or pain at I.V. site • Pain during infusion • Possible blanching if vasospasm occurs • Red skin over vein during infusion • Rapidly developing signs of phlebitis	• Solution with high or low pH or high osmolarity, such as 40 mEq/liter of potassium chloride; phenytoin; and some antibiotics (vancomycin and nafcillin)	• Slow the flow rate. • Try using an electronic flow device to achieve a steady flow. *Prevention:* • Dilute solutions before administration. For example, give antibiotics in 250-ml solution rather than 100 ml. If drug has low pH, ask pharmacist if drug can be buffered with sodium bicarbonate. (Refer to hospital policies.) • If long-term therapy of irritating drug is planned, ask doctor to use central I.V. line.
Severed catheter • Leakage from catheter shaft	• Catheter inadvertently cut by scissors • Reinsertion of needle into catheter	• If broken part is visible, attempt to retrieve it. If unsuccessful, notify doctor. • If portion of catheter enters bloodstream, place tourniquet above I.V. site to prevent progression of broken portion. • Notify doctor and radiology department. • Document patient's condition and your interventions. *Prevention:* • Don't use scissors around I.V. site. • Never reinsert needle into catheter. • Remove unsuccessfully inserted catheter and needle together.

(continued)

COMPLICATIONS

Risks of peripheral I.V. therapy *(continued)*

SIGNS AND SYMPTOMS	POSSIBLE CAUSES	NURSING INTERVENTIONS
Local complications *(continued)*		
Hematoma • Tenderness at veni-puncture site • Area around site bruised • Inability to advance or flush I.V. line	• Vein punctured through other wall at time of venipuncture • Leakage of blood from needle displace-ment	• Remove venipuncture device. • Apply pressure and warm soaks to affected area. • Recheck for bleeding. • Document patient's condition and your interventions. *Prevention:* • Choose a vein that can accommo-date size of venipuncture device. • Release tourniquet as soon as suc-cessful insertion is achieved.
Venous spasm • Pain along vein • Flow rate sluggish when clamp completely open • Blanched skin over vein	• Severe vein irritation from irritating drugs or fluids • Administration of cold fluids or blood • Very rapid flow rate (with fluids at room temperature)	• Apply warm soaks over vein and surrounding area. • Slow flow rate. *Prevention:* • Use blood warmer for blood or packed red blood cells.
Vasovagal reaction • Sudden collapse of vein during venipunc-ture • Sudden pallor accom-panied by sweating, faintness, dizziness, and nausea • Decreased blood pressure	• Vasospasm from anxiety or pain	• Lower head of bed. • Have patient take deep breaths. • Check vital signs. *Prevention:* • Prepare patient adequately for ther-apy to relieve his anxiety. • Use local anesthetic to prevent pain of venipuncture.
Thrombosis • Painful, reddened, and swollen vein • Sluggish or stopped I.V. flow	• Injury to endothelial cells of vein wall, al-lowing platelets to ad-here and thrombus to form	• Remove venipuncture device: restart infusion in opposite limb if possible. • Apply warm soaks. • Watch for I.V. therapy related infec-tion: thrombi provide an excellent en-vironment for bacterial growth. *Prevention:* • Use proper venipuncture techniques to reduce injury to vein.
Thrombophlebitis • Severe discomfort • Reddened, swollen, and hardened vein	• Thrombosis and in-flammation	• Same as for thrombosis. *Prevention:* • Check site frequently. Remove veni-puncture device at first sign of red-ness and tenderness.

Risks of peripheral I.V. therapy   *(continued)*

SIGNS AND SYMPTOMS	POSSIBLE CAUSES	NURSING INTERVENTIONS
Local complications *(continued)*		
Nerve, tendon, or ligament damage		
• Extreme pain (similar to electrical shock when nerve is punctured) • Numbness and muscle contraction • Delayed effects including paralysis, numbness, and deformity	• Improper venipuncture technique, resulting in injury to surrounding nerves, tendons, or ligaments • Tight taping or improper splinting with armboard	• Stop procedure. *Prevention:* • Don't repeatedly penetrate tissues with venipuncture device. • Don't apply excessive pressure when taping or encircle limb with tape. • Pad armboards and pad tape securing armboard if possible.
Systemic complications		
Circulatory overload		
• Discomfort • Neck vein engorgement • Respiratory distress • Increased blood pressure • Crackles • Increased difference between fluid intake and output	• Roller clamp loosened to allow run-on infusion • Flow rate too rapid • Miscalculation of fluid requirements	• Raise the head of the bed. • Administer oxygen as needed. • Notify doctor. • Administer medications (probably furosemide) as ordered. *Prevention:* • Use pump, controller, or rate minder for elderly or compromised patients. • Recheck calculations of fluid requirements. • Monitor infusion frequently.
Systemic infection (septicemia or bacteremia)		
• Fever, chills, and malaise for no apparent reason • Contaminated I.V. site, usually with no visible signs of infection at site	• Failure to maintain aseptic technique during insertion or site care • Severe phlebitis, which can set up ideal conditions for organism growth • Poor taping that permits venipuncture device to move, which can introduce organisms into bloodstream • Prolonged indwelling time of venipuncture device • Immunocompromised patient	• Notify doctor. • Administer medications as prescribed. • Culture site and device. • Monitor vital signs. *Prevention:* • Use scrupulous aseptic technique when handling solutions and tubings, inserting venipuncture device, and discontinuing infusion. • Secure all connections. • Change I.V. solutions, tubing, and venipuncture device at recommended times. • Use I.V. filters.

(continued)

COMPLICATIONS

Risks of peripheral I.V. therapy *(continued)*

SIGNS AND SYMPTOMS	POSSIBLE CAUSES	NURSING INTERVENTIONS
Systemic complications *(continued)*		
Air embolism • Respiratory distress • Unequal breath sounds • Weak pulse • Increased central venous pressure • Decreased blood pressure • Loss of consciousness	• Solution container empty • Solution container empties, and added container pushes air down line	• Discontinue infusion. • Place patient in Trendelenburg's position to allow air to enter right atrium and disperse via pulmonary artery. • Administer oxygen. • Notify doctor. • Document patient's condition and your interventions. *Prevention:* • Purge tubing of air completely before infusion. • Use air-detection device on pump or air-eliminating filter proximal to I.V. site. • Secure connections.
Allergic reaction • Itching • Tearing eyes and runny nose • Bronchospasm • Wheezing • Urticarial rash • Edema at I.V. site • Anaphylactic reaction (may occur within minutes or up to 1 hour after exposure), including flushing, chills, anxiety, agitation, generalized itching, palpitations, paresthesia, throbbing in ears, wheezing, coughing, convulsions, and cardiac arrest	• Allergens such as medications	• If reaction occurs, stop infusion immediately. • Maintain patent airway. • Notify doctor. • Administer antihistaminic steroid, anti-inflammatory, and antipyretic drugs, as ordered. • Give 0.2 to 0.5 ml of 1:1,000 aqueous epinephrine subcutaneously. Repeat at 3-minute intervals and as needed. • Administer cortisone if ordered. *Prevention:* • Obtain patient's allergy history. Be aware of cross-allergies. • Assist with test dosing. • Monitor patient carefully during first 15 minutes of administration of a new drug.

notified, and treatment given. If your patient develops a severe infusion-related problem — for instance, vesicant extravasation, circulatory compromise, a skin tear, fluid overload, or a severe allergic reaction — fill out an incident report. For legal purposes, document the details of the complication as well as medical and nursing interventions.

Discontinuing the infusion

To stop the infusion, first clamp the I.V. line. Then proceed to remove the venipuncture device as painlessly as possible, using aseptic technique. After putting on gloves, lift the tape from the skin to expose the insertion site. You don't need to remove the tape or dressing as long as you can peel it back to expose the venipuncture device and skin.

Be careful to avoid manipulating the device in the skin to prevent skin organisms from entering the bloodstream. Moving the device may also cause pain, especially if the insertion site is phlebitic.

Apply a sterile 2″ × 2″ dressing directly over the insertion site. Then quickly remove the device and the tape from the skin. (Never use an alcohol pad to clean the site when discontinuing an infusion; this may cause bleeding and a burning sensation.) Maintain direct pressure on the I.V. site for 1 to 2 minutes. Then tape a dressing over it, being careful not to encircle the limb. If possible, hold the limb upright for about 5 minutes to decrease venous pressure.

Tell the patient to restrict his activity for about 10 minutes and to leave the site dressing in place for at least 8 hours. If he feels lingering tenderness at the I.V. site, apply warm packs or have him place the site under warm running water for 5 minutes several times a day.

Dispose of the used venipuncture device, tubing, and solution containers in a receptacle for blood products.

Document the time of removal, the catheter length and integrity, and the condition of the site. Also record how the patient tolerated the procedure and any nursing interventions.

Suggested readings

Delaney, C.W., and Lauer, M.L. *Intravenous Therapy: A Guide to Quality Care.* Philadelphia: J.B. Lippincott, 1988.

LaRocca, J.C., and Otto, S.E. *Pocket Guide to Intravenous Therapy.* St. Louis: C.V. Mosby Co., 1989.

Millam, D.A. "Managing Complications of I.V. Therapy," *Nursing88* 18(3):34-43, March 1988.

Millam, D.A. "Tips for Improving Your Venipuncture Techniques," *Nursing87* 17(6):46-49, June 1987.

Nursing90 I.V. Drug Handbook. Springhouse, Pa.: Springhouse Corp., 1990.

Plumer, A. *Principles and Practice of Intravenous Therapy,* 4th ed. Boston: Little, Brown & Co., 1987.

3

CENTRAL VENOUS THERAPY

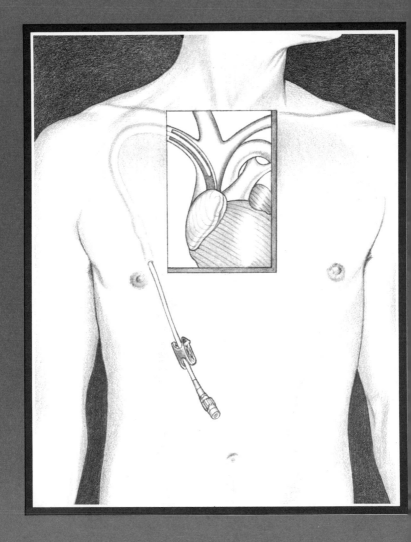

At one time, only certain patients in intensive care and specialty units received central venous (CV) therapy. But today, patients in any unit as well as those at home can benefit from this therapy. To give these patients the care they require, you must understand the basic principles and procedures of CV therapy, including the nursing assessment and interventions you'll need to perform.

This chapter helps you acquire the knowledge and skills you need by providing an overview of CV therapy, including its indications and its advantages and disadvantages. The chapter then explains how to prepare the patient for catheter insertion, choose the equipment, and select the best insertion site. You'll also learn how to assist with catheter insertion and to maintain and discontinue CV therapy.

Basics of CV therapy

Central venous therapy refers to the use of the body's major veins, such as the superior vena cava and the inferior vena cava. Venous return from the head, neck, and arms enters the superior vena cava through the subclavian vein and the internal and external jugular veins and flows into the right atrium. The inferior vena cava carries blood from the legs and the abdomen into the right atrium.

When the CV catheter is positioned correctly, its tip lies in the superior vena cava, inferior vena cava, or the right atrium — that is, in the CV circulation. Blood flows unimpeded around the tip, allowing the rapid infusion of large amounts of fluids directly into the circulation.

A variation of CV therapy, peripheral CV therapy involves the insertion of a catheter in a peripheral vein instead of a major vein, but the catheter tip still lies in the CV circulation. For instance, a catheter entering the basilic vein travels into the superior vena cava, via the subclavian vein and the innominate vein. New catheters have longer needles and smaller lumens, facilitating this procedure.

CV therapy proves extremely helpful in emergencies or when a patient's peripheral veins are inaccessible. And because fluids are rapidly diluted by the CV circulation, highly osmolar or caustic fluids can be infused.

A doctor may also order CV therapy when a patient needs an infusion of a large volume of fluid or when a patient requires long-term venous access.

Advantages and disadvantages
CV therapy offers several advantages, including access to the central veins, which allows for rapid infusion of large amounts of fluids, infusion of medications, and a means to draw blood samples and measure central venous pressure (CVP), an important indicator of circulatory function. Because CV therapy eliminates the need for repeated venipunctures, it decreases the patient's anxiety while preserving (or restoring) the peripheral veins. It also lessens the chance of vein irritation from infusing caustic substances.

As with any invasive procedure, however, CV therapy also has its drawbacks. It increases the risk of complications — such as pneumothorax, sepsis, thrombus formation, and vessel and adjacent organ perforation — all life-threatening conditions. Also, the CV catheter decreases patient mobility, requires

Teaching your patient about CV catheter insertion

Before you teach a patient about central venous (CV) catheter insertion, find out what he knows about the procedure and reinforce any earlier explanation of its goals. Then cover the points in the checklist below.

☐ Teach the patient to perform the Valsalva maneuver, and have him demonstrate it at least twice.

☐ Explain the importance of lying still and maintaining proper position during the procedure.

☐ Mention that he'll be wearing sterile drapes and possibly a mask during catheter insertion.

☐ Tell him to expect a stinging sensation during administration of the local anesthetic and pressure during catheter insertion.

☐ Explain that the CV catheter will be anchored in place with sutures after insertion.

☐ Mention the need for frequent dressing changes.

☐ Describe any motion restrictions he must observe.

☐ Tell him to report if his dressing becomes wet or loose, if the tubing becomes disconnected, if the catheter becomes dislodged, or if he feels pain, pressure, shortness of breath, or light-headedness.

more time and skill to insert than a peripheral I.V. catheter, and costs more than a peripheral I.V. catheter.

Preparing for catheter insertion and infusion

Before the CV catheter is inserted, you need to prepare the patient

both physically and mentally. Preparation for catheter insertion also involves choosing and collecting the infusion equipment and selecting an insertion site for the CV catheter. Typically, the doctor will make these choices after discussing the options with you.

Preparing the patient

Before therapy begins, make sure the patient understands the procedure, its benefit to him, and what's expected of him during and after the catheter insertion. Although the primary responsibility for explaining the procedure and its goals rests with the doctor, you must be prepared to supplement the explanation. You'll also need to allay the patient's fears and answer questions about movement restrictions, cosmetic concerns, and management regimens. Your accurate and thorough patient teaching helps make therapy successful. (See *Teaching your patient about CV catheter insertion*.)

Explaining the procedure. Ask your patient if he's ever received I.V. therapy before, particularly CV therapy. Evaluate his learning capabilities, and adjust your teaching technique accordingly. For example, use appropriate language to describe the procedure to a child. Also, ask the parents to help you phrase the procedure in terms their child understands. If time and resources permit, use pictures and physical models to enhance your teaching.

If the catheter insertion will take place at the bedside, explain that sterile procedures require the staff to wear gowns, masks, and gloves. Tell your patient he may need to wear a mask as well. If time allows, let your patient try on the mask—especially if he's a child.

To minimize the patient's anxiety and discomfort, explain how he'll be positioned during the procedure. If the subclavian or jugular vein will be used, he'll be in the Trendelenburg position for at least a short period, and a towel may be placed under his back between the scapulae. Reassure him that he won't be in this position longer than necessary, but stress the position's importance for dilating the veins, which aids insertion and helps prevent air embolism.

Warn him to expect a stinging sensation from the local anesthetic and a feeling of pressure during the catheter insertion. Also explain any other tests that may be done. For example, some doctors obtain a venogram before the catheter insertion to check the status of the vessels, especially if the catheter is intended for long-term use. After CV catheter insertion, blood samples are often drawn to establish baseline coagulation profiles, and a chest X-ray is always done to confirm catheter placement.

Explaining care measures. Teach the patient the Valsalva maneuver and have him demonstrate it to you at least twice. Explain that because this maneuver helps prevent air embolism, he'll need to perform it now and in the future — whenever the catheter is open to the air. This training becomes especially important when the patient is taking care of his catheter at home.

Whether catheter insertion takes place in the operating room or at the bedside, the patient-teaching concepts are the same. For an operating room procedure, however, elaborate on preoperative and postoperative procedures and care.

If the catheter will be in place over a long period or will be managed at home, you'll need to explain thoroughly all care procedures, such as changing the dressing and flushing the catheter. Ask your patient to demonstrate the various procedures, and include other family members, as appropriate. A home-therapy coordinator or discharge planner should also get in touch with the home-therapy patient to coordinate teaching and follow-up assessments before and after catheter insertion.

Obtaining consent. Most hospitals require an informed consent before any invasive procedure. The doctor obtains the consent and, most times, you'll be responsible for witnessing the patient's signature. Tell the patient he'll be asked to sign a consent form and explain what this means. (The consent procedure is the same as for surgery.) Before the patient signs, make sure he understands the procedure. If he has concerns or questions, delay signing until you or the doctor clarifies the explanations and the patient shows he understands.

In an emergency, the consent form can be signed by the next of kin, or administrative approval may be granted. In either case, you should still teach the patient about the therapy — even if the teaching occurs after the catheter is in place.

Selecting the equipment
The CV catheter selected for a patient depends on the type of therapy he needs. The catheter and its insertion site, in turn, affect the selection of other infusion equipment. Many CV lines are maintained as intermittent infusion devices (heparin locks), with solutions given at designated times followed by a flush, usually with heparin or saline solution. The flushing procedures

and amounts differ with the type of catheter used.

Choosing the catheter. CV catheters come in three basic types: over-the-needle, through-the-needle, and over-a-guidewire (the most commonly used). All three are made of polyurethane, polyvinylchloride (PVC), or silicone rubber (Silastic). Usually, catheters made of the first two materials are designed for short-term use, while those made of silicone rubber are designed for long-term use.

A catheter's properties and potential complications, in light of the patient's needs, also determine the selection. For example, a patient with a long history of I.V. drug abuse who requires volume replacement after a gunshot wound wouldn't be a candidate for a peripheral CV catheter. Repeated I.V. drug injections may have left his peripheral vessels sclerosed or tortuous. And since this emergency requires immediate short-term therapy, the patient wouldn't be a candidate for a Hickman catheter, either. Instead, the doctor may choose a single-lumen or multilumen PVC catheter, inserted via the internal jugular or subclavian vein.

• *Short-term use.* Catheters designed for short-term use include single-lumen or multilumen catheters made of polyurethane or PVC. Single-lumen catheters have only one opening, allowing the administration of only one solution at a time. Multilumen catheters allow the administration of more than one solution at a time, without regard for compatibility. The size of their internal lumens varies, but the most commonly used catheter has three lumens, a 16G distal lumen, an 18G proximal lumen, and an 18G medial lumen. The distal lumen is used to monitor CVP.

The lumens open into the central vein at approximately ¾″ (2-cm) intervals. The catheters are slightly stiff, allowing for speedier insertion over a guidewire, but also increasing the potential for vessel irritation and rupture from patient movement.

Catheter movement also increases the risk of infection and thrombus formation at the insertion site. The movement may allow surface organisms to migrate into the site and may also cause the formation of a thrombus that could act as a protein-rich medium for even more bacterial growth. Because of these problems, short-term catheters are not meant for prolonged therapy. The Intravenous Nurses Society (INS) recommends these catheters be changed every 3 to 7 days.

• *Long-term use.* Catheters designed for long-term use are more flexible and are usually made of silicone rubber. This material is much less thrombogenic than polyurethane or PVC because it's more physiologically compatible. Since silicone is more flexible, however, insertion may be more difficult.

Insertion is usually performed in the operating room, through a cutdown procedure in which the vein is isolated and the catheter is inserted directly. Once the catheter tip is in the central vein, the remaining portion is placed into the subcutaneous tissue and threaded (tunneled) 1¼″ to 2″ (3 to 5 cm) to an exit site where it surfaces outside the skin. The catheter may be cut to size during the procedure to prevent excess length on the outside. Just before the point where the catheter exits the skin, the doctor positions a Dacron cuff. (See *Identifying CV catheter pathways.*) Granulation tissue forms around the cuff in about 2 weeks, helping

Identifying CV catheter pathways

Usually, a central venous (CV) catheter is inserted into the subclavian vein or the internal jugular vein. The catheter may terminate in the superior vena cava or in the right atrium. The illustrations below show several common pathways of the CV catheter.

This CV catheter, inserted into the subclavian vein, terminates in the superior vena cava.

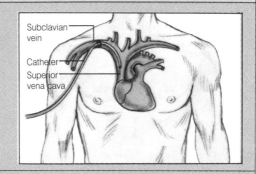

Inserted into the subclavian vein, this CV catheter extends to the right atrium.

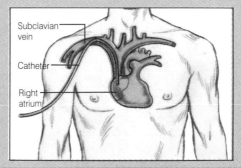

This CV catheter enters the internal jugular vein and terminates in the superior vena cava.

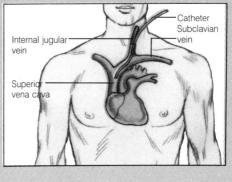

(continued)

Identifying CV catheter pathways *(continued)*

This CV catheter, peripherally inserted into the basilic vein, terminates in the superior vena cava.

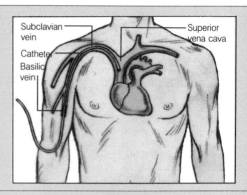

Subclavian vein
Catheter
Basilic vein
Superior vena cava

This CV catheter enters the subclavian vein and terminates in the superior vena cava. Note that the catheter tunnels (shown by broken line) from the insertion site, through the subcutaneous tissue, to an exit site on the skin. Also note how the position of the Dacron cuff helps hold the catheter in place.

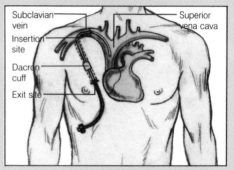

Subclavian vein
Insertion site
Dacron cuff
Exit site
Superior vena cava

secure the catheter in place and acting as a barrier to organism migration.

Examples of silicone rubber long-term devices include the Hickman, Broviac, and Groshong catheters. The Groshong differs from the Hickman and Broviac catheters in that it has a closed end with a two-way pressure-sensitive valve proximal to the end. The valve opens with positive pressure to allow fluid infusion and opens with negative pressure to allow blood withdrawal. The catheter remains closed with neutral pressure, decreasing the risk of air embolism and eliminating the need for heparin flushes. (See

Nurse's guide to CV catheters.)
• *Implantable infusion ports.* Another device, an implantable infusion port consists of catheter tubing attached to an infusion port, which has a self-sealing septum. The infusion port is implanted in a pocket in the subcutaneous tissue, using local anesthesia. Its catheter tunnels to a central vein leading into the right atrium.

Choosing the infusion equipment.
Infusion equipment typically includes I.V. solution and an administration set with tubing. The equipment may also include an infusion pump and a drip controller.

Nurse's guide to CV catheters

Central venous (CV) catheters differ in their design, composition, and indications for use. This chart outlines the advantages, disadvantages, and nursing considerations for several commonly used catheters.

CATHETER DESCRIPTION AND INDICATIONS	ADVANTAGES AND DISADVANTAGES	NURSING CONSIDERATIONS
Short-term, single-lumen catheter *Description:* • Polyvinylchloride (PVC) or polyurethane. • Approximately 8″ (20.3 cm) long. • Lumen gauge varies. *Indications:* • Short-term CV access. • Emergency access. • Patient who needs only one lumen.	*Advantages:* • Easily inserted at bedside. • Easily removed. • Stiffness aids central venous pressure (CVP) monitoring. *Disadvantages:* • Limited functions. • PVC is thrombogenic. • PVC irritates inner lumen of vessel. • Needs to be changed every 3 to 7 days.	• Minimize patient motion. • Assess frequently for signs of infection and clot formation. 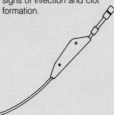
Short-term, multilumen catheter *Description:* • PVC or polyurethane. • Double, triple, or quadruple lumens exiting at ¾″ (2-cm) intervals. • Lumen gauges vary. *Indications:* • Short-term CV access. • Patient with limited insertion sites who requires multiple infusions.	*Advantages:* • See single-lumen catheter. • Allows infusion of multiple solutions through the same catheter – even incompatible solutions. *Disadvantages:* • See single-lumen catheter.	• Know gauge and purpose of each lumen. • Use the same lumen for the same task, for example, total parenteral nutrition (TPN) or blood sampling. 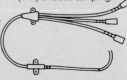
Groshong catheter *Description:* • Silicone rubber. • Approximately 35″ (88.9 cm) long. • Closed end with pressure-sensitive two-way valve. • Dacron cuff. • Available with single or double lumen. *Indications:* • Long-term CV access. • Patient with heparin allergy.	*Advantages:* • Less thrombogenic. • Pressure-sensitive two-way valve eliminates frequent heparin flushes. • Dacron cuff anchors catheter and prevents bacterial migration. *Disadvantages:* • Requires surgical insertion. • Tears and kinks easily. • Blunt end makes it difficult to clear substances from its tip.	• Two surgical sites require dressing after insertion. • Handle catheter gently. • Check the external portion frequently for kinks or leaks. • Repair kit is available. • Remember to flush with enough saline solution to clear catheter, especially after drawing or administering blood.

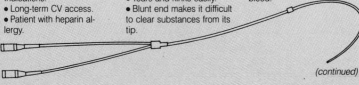

(continued)

Nurse's guide to CV catheters *(continued)*

CATHETER DESCRIPTION AND INDICATIONS	ADVANTAGES AND DISADVANTAGES	NURSING CONSIDERATIONS
Hickman catheter *Description:* • Silicone rubber. • Approximately 35" long. • Open end with clamp. • Dacron cuff 11¾" (30 cm) from hub. • Single-lumen or multilumen. *Indications:* • Long-term CV access. • Home therapy.	*Advantages:* • Less thrombogenic. • Dacron cuff prevents excess motion and organism migration. • Clamps eliminate need for Valsalva maneuver. *Disadvantages:* • Requires surgical insertion. • Open end. • Requires doctor for removal. • Tears and kinks easily.	• Two surgical sites require dressing after insertion. • Handle catheter gently. • Observe frequently for kinks or tears. • Repair kit is available. • Clamp catheter any time it becomes disconnected or open, using nonserrated clamp. 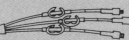
Broviac catheter *Description:* • Identical to Hickman except smaller inner lumen. *Indications:* • Long-term CV access. • Patient with small central vessels (pediatric, elderly).	*Advantages:* • Smaller lumen. *Disadvantages:* • Small lumen may limit its uses. • Single lumen.	• Check hospital policy before drawing or administering blood or blood products. 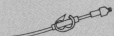
Hickman/Broviac catheter *Description:* • Hickman and Broviac catheters in one catheter. *Indications:* • Long-term CV access. • Patient who needs multiple infusions.	*Advantages:* • Double-lumen Hickman catheter allows sampling and administration of blood. • Broviac lumen delivers I.V. fluids, including TPN. *Disadvantages:* • See Hickman catheter.	• Know purpose and function of each lumen. • Label lumens to prevent confusion. 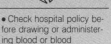
Long-line catheter *Description:* • Peripherally inserted central catheter (PICC). • Silicone rubber. • 20" (50.8 cm) long; available in 16G, 18G, and 20G. *Indications:* • Long-term CV access. • Patient with poor central access. • Patient at risk for fatal complications from central insertion. • Patient who needs CV access but faces or has had head and neck surgery.	*Advantages:* • Peripherally inserted. • Easily inserted at bedside with minimal complications. • May be inserted by trained registered nurse in some states. *Disadvantages:* • Catheter may occlude smaller peripheral vessels. • May be difficult to keep immobile. • Single lumen. • Long path to CV circulation.	• Check frequently for signs of phlebitis and thrombus formation. • Insert catheter above the antecubital fossa. • Use armboard if necessary. • Catheter may alter CVP measurements. 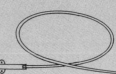 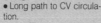

Expect to use an infusion pump any time positive pressure is required, for example, when solutions are administered through a CV line at low flow rates or during intra-arterial infusion. Some hospitals use drip controllers for CV therapy, which permits infusion at a lower pressure. Drip controllers are used most often with infants and children, who could suffer serious complications from high-pressure infusion.

Selecting the insertion site

The insertion site will vary, depending on the catheter that's being used and the patient's anatomy. The doctor must consider these factors as well as vessel integrity and accessibility; the patient's age; the length of the therapy; probable complications; any history of previous neck or chest surgery, such as mastectomy; and the presence of chest trauma.

Scar tissue from previous surgery or trauma may prohibit access to the vessels or make threading the catheter difficult. If the patient is facing surgery in the area, another site should be chosen—perhaps, a peripheral site such as the brachial vein or a central site on the side of the body unaffected by surgery. If the patient has a tracheostomy, the internal or external jugular site should be avoided because the tracheostomy tapes come too close to these insertion sites, predisposing the patient to infection and possibly causing the catheter to dislodge.

Another site consideration is the location of the lung apices. In patients on mechanical ventilation, especially positive end-expiratory pressure, intrathoracic pressures increase, possibly elevating the lung apices and increasing the chance of lung puncture and pneumothorax.

Patients with chronic obstructive pulmonary disease also have displaced lung apices, so sites other than those in the thorax should be considered.

Practical considerations also play a role in site selection. For example, a home-therapy patient with a peripheral CV catheter would have only one hand with which to work. And a woman with a long-term catheter that exits near her brassiere straps would have a limited choice of clothing.

Being aware of the catheter's insertion and termination points helps keep you alert for potential complications, such as thrombosis, catheter displacement, or infection at the sites. Veins commonly used as CV insertion sites include the subclavian, internal and external jugular, and cephalic. The femoral and brachial veins may be used, but this occurs rarely. (See *Comparing CV insertion sites,* page 84.)

Subclavian vein. The most common insertion site, the subclavian vein affords easy access and a short, direct route to the superior vena cava and the CV circulation. Because it's a large vein with a high-volume blood flow, it's less apt to be associated with thrombus formation and vessel irritation. The subclavian site also allows the greatest patient mobility after insertion. Plus, you'll find that the dressing will stay in place.

When using this site, the doctor inserts the catheter into the vein percutaneously (through the skin and into the vessel with one puncture), threading it into the superior vena cava. This technique requires a venous puncture close to the apex of the lung and major vessels of the thorax. As the catheter enters the skin between the clavicle and first

Comparing CV insertion sites

The chart below lists the most common insertion sites for a central venous (CV) catheter and the advantages and disadvantages of each.

SITE	ADVANTAGES	DISADVANTAGES
Subclavian vein	• Easy access • Easy to keep dressing in place • High flow rate, reducing thrombus formation	• Proximity to subclavian artery • Difficult to control bleeding • Increased risk of pneumothorax
Internal jugular vein	• Short, direct route to right atrium • Catheter stability, resulting in less movement with respiration • Decreased risk of pneumothorax	• Proximity to the common carotid artery • Difficult to keep dressing in place • Proximity to the trachea
External jugular vein	• Easy access, especially in children • Decreased risk of pneumothorax or arterial puncture	• Less direct route • Lower flow rate, increasing risk of thrombus • Difficult to keep dressing in place • Tortuous vein, especially in elderly patients
Cephalic, basilic veins	• Least risk of major complications • Easy to keep dressing in place	• May require a cutdown • May prove difficult to locate antecubital fossa in obese patients • Difficult to keep elbow immobile, especially in children

rib, the doctor directs the needle toward the angle of Louis, under the clavicle. The doctor may have difficulty with the procedure if the patient moves during insertion or has a chest deformity or poor posture.

Internal jugular vein. An insertion site often used in children (not infants), the internal jugular vein provides easy access in small patients. The right internal jugular vein provides a more direct route to the superior vena cava than the

left internal jugular vein. However, its proximity to the common carotid artery can lead to serious complications, such as uncontrolled hemorrhage, emboli, or impedance to flow if the carotid artery is punctured during catheter insertion. Puncture of the carotid artery can cause irreversible brain damage.

The use of the internal jugular vein also has other drawbacks. For example, it limits patient movement and may be considered a poor choice for home therapy because of cosmetic considerations. Because f the location of the internal jugular vein, it's also difficult to keep a dressing in place.

Peripheral veins. Among the peripheral veins most commonly used as insertion sites are the cephalic, basilic, and external jugular. Because they're far away from major thoracic organs and vessels, peripheral veins are associated with fewer traumatic complications upon insertion. However, peripheral veins are often associated with vessel irritation because the tight fit of the catheter in the smaller vessel allows for only minimal blood flow around the catheter. Catheter movement may irritate the inner lumen or occlude it altogether, resulting in blood stasis and thrombus formation.

Peripheral sites also limit patient mobility because they usually exit the skin at the antecubital space. Inserting the catheter above the antecubital space increases patient mobility and avoids kinking, although you may find it difficult to see the veins here.

The most commonly used catheter for peripheral CV therapy is the peripherally inserted central catheter (PICC). In many states, registered nurses are allowed to insert this catheter.

• *Cephalic and basilic veins.* Although the cephalic vein is more accessible than the basilic vein, its sharp angle makes it more difficult to thread. The larger, straighter basilic vein is usually the preferred insertion site.

• *External jugular vein.* Sometimes considered a peripheral CV insertion site, the external jugular vein presents few complications. Threading a catheter into the superior vena cava may prove difficult, however, because of the sharp angle encoun-

tered upon entering the subclavian vein. For this reason, the catheter tip may remain in the external jugular vein. This placement allows high-volume infusions, but it makes CVP measurement inaccurate.

External jugular veins should not be used to administer highly caustic medications because blood flow around the tip of the catheter may not be strong enough to sufficiently dilute the solutions as they enter the vein.

Assisting with catheter insertion

Before the doctor inserts the catheter, you need to set up the infusion equipment, prepare the insertion site, and position the patient. You'll follow the same basic procedures whether the insertion is done at the bedside or in the operating room, although the specific steps may vary.

After the catheter has been inserted, your primary responsibilities are to monitor the patient and start administering the therapy. You'll also need to apply a dressing to the insertion site and document your interventions, according to your hospital's policy.

Setting up the equipment
To set up the equipment, you need to attach the tubing to the solution container, prime the tubing with the solution, fill the syringes with saline or heparin flush solution, and prime and calibrate any pressure monitoring setups. All priming must be done using strict aseptic technique, and all tubing must be free of air. After you've primed the tubing,

recheck all the connections to see that they're tight. Make sure all open ends are covered with sealed caps.

If you're assisting with an insertion at the patient's bedside, you should first collect the necessary equipment. Most hospitals use preassembled disposable trays that include the CV catheter. Although most trays include the necessary equipment, be sure to check. If you don't have a preassembled tray, gather the following items: a linen-saver pad; scissors; povidone-iodine solution; sterile gauze pads; a solution of 70% alcohol or hydrogen peroxide, if ordered; local anesthetic; small syringe with 25G needle for introduction of anesthetic; sterile syringe for blood samples; sterile towels or drapes; suture material; sterile dressing; and the CV catheter.

You'll need masks, gowns, and gloves for everyone participating in the insertion. You may also need such protection for the patient, especially if there's a risk of site contamination from the oral secretions of a patient who is unable to cooperate. Obtain extra syringes and blood sample containers, if the doctor orders venous blood samples to be drawn during the procedure.

Preparing the site
After you've assembled the equipment, position the patient and make him as comfortable as possible. The patient will be in the Trendelenburg position (for insertion in the subclavian or internal jugular veins) during the procedure because it distends his neck and thoracic veins, making them more visible and accessible. Filling the veins also lessens the chance of air emboli because venous pressure is higher than atmospheric pressure.

If the subclavian vein will be used, place a rolled towel or blanket between the patient's scapulae. This allows for more direct access and may prevent puncture of the lung apex or adjacent vessels. If a jugular vein will be used, place a rolled blanket under the opposite shoulder to extend the neck and make anatomic landmarks more visible.

Now, prepare the insertion site using the following steps:
• Place a linen-saver pad under the site to prevent soiling the bed.
• Make sure the skin is free of hair; the follicles can harbor microorganisms. Infection-control practitioners and the INS recommend clipping the hair close to the skin rather than shaving. Shaving may cause skin irritation and create multiple small open wounds, increasing the risk of infection. (If the doctor orders the area to be shaved, try to shave it the evening before; this allows minor skin irritations to partially heal before irritating cleaning substances are applied.) After you remove the hair, rinse the skin with saline solution to remove hair clippings. You may find that you also need to wash the skin with soap and water before the actual skin prep to remove surface dirt and body oils.
• Ensure each person participating in the catheter insertion dons gowns, gloves, and masks.
• Prep the site with povidone-iodine solution, using a sterile gauze pad. If the patient is allergic to iodine, you may use a solution of 70% alcohol. Use a circular motion to prep the skin, starting at the insertion site and gradually making wider circles with each motion. Don't wipe the same area twice and be sure to discard each gauze pad

fter each complete cycle. (The
octor may prep the site in an emer-
ency.)

After the site is prepped, the
octor will place sterile drapes
round it, and possibly around the
atient's face, as well. (This would
ake the patient's mask unneces-
ary.) The drapes should provide a
ork area at least as large as the
ength of the catheter or guidewire.
f the patient's face is draped, you
an help ease his anxiety by uncov-
ring his eyes.

ssisting with the procedure

uring the insertion, you may be
sponsible for handing equipment
nd supplies to the doctor, such
s the local anesthetic. Expect to
pen sterile packages of syringes,
ipe the tops of medication vials,
nd invert the vials so the doctor
an withdraw the medications.

If the doctor wants venous blood
amples after the catheter is in-
erted, he'll obtain them before con-
ecting the I.V. tubing and starting
ne infusion. Hand the doctor a
terile syringe that's large enough
o hold all of the needed blood.
hen, place the blood in the proper
ample container. Each time the
atheter hub is open to air — when
ne syringe is changed, for
nstance — tell the patient to perform
ne Valsalva maneuver to decrease
ne risk of air embolism.

Monitoring the patient

fter the catheter has been inserted,
nonitor the patient for complica-
ions. Make sure you tailor your as-
essment and interventions to the
articular catheter insertion site.
or example, if the site is close to
najor thoracic organs, as is a sub-
lavian or internal jugular site,
ou should closely monitor the pa-
ient's respiratory status, watching

for dyspnea, shortness of breath,
and sudden chest pain.

Because the insertion may cause
arrhythmias if the catheter enters
the right ventricle and irritates the
ventricular wall, you should also
monitor the patient's cardiac status.
(Arrhythmias will usually abate as
the catheter is withdrawn.) If the
patient isn't attached to a cardiac
monitor, you should palpate his
radial artery to detect any rhythm
irregularities.

Initiating therapy

Connect the I.V. tubing or intermittent cap to the catheter hub. If
the line will be used for infusion,
run an isotonic fluid at a rate no
greater than 20 ml/hour until the
catheter placement has been confirmed by an X-ray. The proximal
end of the catheter should now rest
on the sterile drape. Maintain sterile
technique until the catheter is sutured in place and a sterile dressing
is placed over the site.

The doctor will use one or two
sutures to secure the catheter to the
skin. Most short-term catheters
have preset tabs to hold the sutures.
Make sure the suturing leaves the
catheter properly positioned outside
the skin; a poor position can make
an airtight dressing difficult or
impossible to apply and may cause
the catheter to kink.

Applying the dressing. After the CV
catheter is in place, apply the
dressing to the insertion site of a
short-term catheter or to the exit
site of a long-term catheter. Remember to keep the site clean and dry
to prevent infection and to keep the
dressing airtight to prevent air
embolism. To apply the dressing,
follow these steps:
• Clean the site with saline solution
or hydrogen peroxide to remove

dried blood, which could harbor microorganisms.

• Now, clean the site with povidone-iodine solution, using the same method as the initial skin prep.

• Place a drop of antibiotic ointment at the site, if hospital policy directs.

• Cover the site with dry, sterile gauze or a transparent semipermeable dressing.

• Seal the dressing with nonporous tape, checking that all edges are well secured. Label the dressing with the date, time, your initials, and the catheter length.

After you apply the dressing, place the patient in a comfortable position and reassess his status. Elevating the head of the bed 45 degrees will help him breathe easier. Remember, X-ray confirmation of catheter placement is always done before infusing any fluids, other than slowly infusing isotonic solutions. After the X-ray confirmation, adjust the flow rate.

Documenting the insertion. Make sure your documentation includes the type of catheter used, the entry or exit site (for a long-term CV catheter), the catheter tip position as confirmed by an X-ray, the patient's tolerance of the procedure, and any blood samples taken. Include this information in the narrative notes and on the I.V. flow sheet, if your hospital uses them.

Some hospitals recommend documenting the length of catheter remaining outside the body so subsequent nurses can compare the measurements, checking for catheter migration. This measurement is not always accurate, however, because some catheters, such as the Hickman, Broviac, and Groshong, may be cut and repaired if they collapse or tear, which would alter the measurement.

Maintaining CV therapy

After the CV infusion begins, your primary responsibility is to maintain it. Among other things, you'll need to change the dressing whenever it becomes moist, loose, or soiled (or at least once every 72 hours). You'll also need to care for the catheter—a task that involves changing the tubing, solution container, and cap, and flushing the catheter. Also, you may be asked to administer a secondary infusion or obtain blood samples.

Maintaining therapy also involves preventing common problems, such as catheter tears and kinks, fluid leaks, and clot formation at the catheter's tip. You may also need to tailor your interventions to meet the requirements of pediatric, elderly, and home-therapy patients. Finally, you must be prepared to manage traumatic complications, such as a pneumothorax, and systemic complications, such as sepsis.

Routine care
Most of the routine care measures you'll perform involve the catheter and its insertion site. These measures include changing the dressing, changing the solution and the tubing, flushing the catheter, changing the cap, and maintaining all connections. You may also perform other routine measures, such as administering a secondary infusion or obtaining blood samples. Throughout the infusion, document your assessment findings and interventions, as hospital policy directs.

Dressing changes. To reduce the risk of infection, always wear gloves, a mask, and a gown when hanging the dressing. Anyone within 10 feet of the patient should also wear a mask, including the patient if he is immunocompromised; if he's not immunocompromised, have him turn his head away from the catheter during the dressing change. (See *Key steps to changing a dressing,* page 90.)

Many hospitals use a preassembled dressing change tray that contains all the necessary equipment. If your hospital doesn't use this type of tray, gather the following equipment: povidone-iodine swabs and ointment, alcohol swabs, sterile 4″ × 4″ gauze pads, 1″ adhesive tape or transparent semipermeable dressing, hydrogen peroxide, sterile gloves and masks, clean gloves, and a bag to dispose the old dressing.

To change the dressing, follow these steps:

Wash your hands thoroughly.

Prepare a sterile field. Open the bag, placing it away from the sterile field but still within reach.

Place the patient in a comfortable position.

Put on clean gloves and remove the old dressing, being careful not to pull the catheter.

Inspect the old dressing for signs of infection. You may want to culture any discharge at the site or on the old dressing. If not, discard the dressing in the bag. Be sure to report an infection to the doctor immediately and to document it in the nurses' notes.

Check the position of the catheter and the insertion site for evidence of infiltration or infection, such as redness, swelling, irritation, tenderness, or drainage.

Put on sterile gloves and clean the skin around the catheter with alcohol or peroxide, wiping outward from the insertion site in a circular manner as you did when preparing the skin. Clean the site with alcohol a total of three times.

• Clean the skin around the site with povidone-iodine, moving outward from the insertion site. Do this three times also. Don't use solutions containing acetone; they may react with some catheters and cause them to disintegrate. Also, make sure the alcohol is completely dry before cleaning with povidone-iodine; otherwise, the combination may cause formation of a tincture of iodine solution, which can cause skin irritation and breakdown.

• Redress the site with sterile 4″ × 4″ gauze pads, and tape the dressing in place. A transparent semipermeable dressing may also be used. If your hospital policy directs, apply povidone-iodine ointment to the insertion site, then cover the site with a 2″ × 2″ sterile gauze pad, followed by a 4″ × 4″ sterile gauze pad. Tape all edges occlusively.

• If the catheter is taped (not sutured) to the skin, carefully replace the soiled tape with sterile tape, using the chevron method. To do so, first cut a strip of tape about ½″ thick and slide it under the catheter, sticky side up. Then, crisscross the tape over the top of the catheter. Finally, place a second strip of tape over the first strip. Be sure the catheter is secure.

• After the site has been dressed, label the dressing with the date, time, and your initials.

• Discard all used items properly; reposition the patient comfortably.

Changing the solution and tubing.
Change the I.V. solution and tubing every 24 hours or as directed by your hospital's policy, maintaining strict aseptic technique. You don't need to wear a mask while perform-

Key steps to changing a dressing

Expect to change your patient's dressing at least every 72 hours, or whenever it becomes soiled, moist, or loose. The following illustrations show three key steps you'll perform.

Wearing clean gloves, remove the old dressing by pulling it toward the exit site of a long-term catheter or toward the insertion site of a short-term catheter. (This technique helps you avoid pulling out the line.) Remove and discard your gloves.

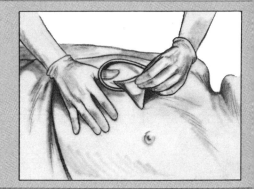

Wearing sterile gloves, clean the skin around the site with an alcohol swab three times. Start at the center and move outward, using a circular motion. Allow the skin to dry and repeat the same cleaning procedure using povidone-iodine solution.

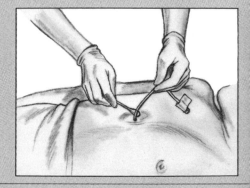

After the solution has dried, cover the site with a dressing, such as the transparent semipermeable dressing shown here.

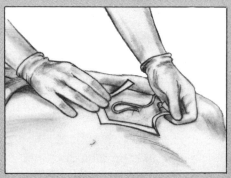

ıg this procedure, unless there's contamination risk (for instance, if ou have an upper respiratory ract infection).

To prevent air embolism, have the atient perform the Valsalva maneuver each time the catheter hub is pen to air. Many hospitals eliminate the need for this by using connecting tubing with a slide lamp between the catheter hub and he I.V. tubing, which allows the .V. tubing to be clamped during hanges.

If possible, change the solution nd tubing at the same time. (You ıay not be able to do this if, for xample, the tubing is damaged or he solution runs out before it's time ɔ change the tubing.)

To change the solution, gather a olution container and an alcohol wab. Then follow these steps:
Wash your hands.
If the container is being replaced, emove the cap and seal, and swab he stopper with alcohol.
Clamp the CV line using a padded lamp to prevent damage to the atheter. Remove the spike and uickly reinsert it into the new botle. Hang the new bottle and adjust he flow rate.

To change the tubing, gather an .V. administration set, a sterile " × 2" gauze pad, adhesive tape, nd hemostat (optional). Then follow hese steps:
Wash your hands.
Place the sterile 2" × 2" gauze ad under the needle or catheter ub to create a sterile field.
Reduce the I.V. flow rate and emove the old spike from the bag. oosely spread the cover from the ew spike over the old spike.
Keep the old spike in an upright osition above the patient's heart nd insert the new spike into the .V. container. Prime the system.

• Instruct the patient to perform the Valsalva maneuver. Quickly disconnect the old tubing from the needle or catheter hub, being careful not to dislodge the venipuncture device. If it's difficult to disconnect, use a hemostat to hold the hub securely while the end of the tubing is twisted and removed. Don't clamp the hemostat shut because the tubing adapter, needle, or catheter hub may crack, requiring a change of equipment and I.V. site.
• Quickly attach the new primed tubing to the venipuncture device, using aseptic technique.
• Adjust the flow to the prescribed rate.
• Label the new tubing with the date and time of change.

To change the tubing and solution simultaneously, follow these steps:
• Wash your hands.
• Hang the new I.V. bag and primed tubing on the I.V. pole.
• Stop the flow in the old tubing.
• Quickly disconnect the old tubing and connect the new tubing, as described above.

Flushing the catheter. To maintain patency, routinely flush the catheter, according to your hospital's policy. If the system is being maintained as a heparin lock and the infusions are intermittent, the flushing procedure will vary according to the hospital's policy, the medication administration schedule, and the type of catheter being used.

Generally, a CV catheter with a two-way valve (Groshong catheter) needs to be flushed with saline solution once a week. All lumens of a multilumen catheter (unless it is a Groshong catheter) must be flushed regularly with heparinized saline solution. (No flushing is needed with a continuous infusion through a single-lumen catheter.)

Most hospitals use a heparinized saline flush solution, available in premixed 10-ml multidose vials. Recommended concentration strengths vary from 10 units of heparin/ml to 1,000 units of heparin/ml. Some hospitals use saline solution instead of heparinized saline solution to flush catheters because research shows heparin isn't always necessary to keep the line open.

The recommended frequency for flushing varies from once every 12 hours to once a week. Most clinicians agree that flushing should be done twice a day for 3 to 4 days postoperatively, and from once a day to 3 times a week after that.

The recommended amount of flushing solution also varies. Most hospitals recommend using 3 to 5 ml of solution to flush the catheter, although some hospitals' policies call for as much as 10 ml of solution. Different catheters require different amounts of solution. For example, the volume capacity for the Hickman catheter is less than 2 ml, while the Broviac catheter has only a 1-ml capacity. The volume capacity will be altered if the catheter is cut to fit the patient.

To flush the catheter, follow these steps:
• Clean the cap with an alcohol swab (using a 70% alcohol solution) and allow it to dry.
• Inject the recommended type and amount of flush solution.
• After flushing, maintain positive pressure by keeping your thumb on the plunger of the syringe while withdrawing the needle. This prevents blood backflow and potential clotting in the line.

Changing the cap. CV catheters used for intermittent infusions have injection caps — short luer-lock devices similar to the heparin lock adapters used for peripheral I.V. infusion therapy. Unlike heparin lock adapters, however, these caps have a small amount of empty space, so you don't have to preflush the cap before connecting it.

The frequency of cap changes varies according to hospital policy and the number of times that the cap is used. Use strict aseptic technique when changing the cap; repeated punctures of the injection port increase the risk of infection. Also, pieces of the rubber stopper may break off after repeated punctures, placing the patient at risk for embolism. To change the cap, follow these steps:
• Clean the connection site with an alcohol or povidone-iodine swab.
• Instruct the patient to perform the Valsalva maneuver while you quickly disconnect the old cap and connect the new cap, using aseptic technique. If the patient can't perform the Valsalva maneuver, use a padded clamp to prevent air from entering the catheter.

Administering secondary fluids. If other fluids will be added to the patient's CV infusion, make sure that solutions running in the same line are compatible. Also check that the connections are well secured with tape.

Secondary I.V. lines are often piggybacked into the cap of a CV catheter instead of being connected directly to the catheter lumen, particularly if the solutions are infusing over a short period (30 minutes). If the infusion is to run over a longer period, remove the cap and attach the tubing via the luerlock connection rather than with a needle through the cap. (This prevents the needle puncture of the catheter, a common problem with Hickman and Broviac catheters.)

Drawing blood. You may receive an order to use the CV catheter to obtain blood samples, especially if the patient has poor peripheral veins. To do so using an evacuated tube, follow these steps:

Wash your hands and put on sterile gloves.

Stop the I.V. infusion and place an injection cap on the lumen of the catheter.

If multiple infusions are running, stop them and wait 1 minute before drawing blood from the catheter. This allows I.V. fluids and medications to be carried away from the catheter, preventing them from becoming mixed with the blood sample you'll be drawing.

Clean the end of the injection cap with antiseptic swabs (povidone-iodine and alcohol).

Place a 5-ml lavender-top evacuated tube into its plastic sleeve. You'll use this tube to collect and discard the filling volume of the catheter, plus an extra 2 to 3 ml. Most studies indicate that about 5 ml is enough blood to discard.

(At some hospitals, the first 5 ml of blood isn't discarded if the patient is scheduled for multiple blood studies. Instead, the blood is infused back into the patient after the sample is drawn.)

Insert the needle into the injection cap of the catheter. The first milliliter may be clear until the blood flows through the catheter.

When blood stops flowing into the tube, remove and discard it, if appropriate.

Use the appropriate evacuated tubes for the ordered blood tests. After you've drawn the necessary blood, flush the catheter with saline solution and resume the infusion. If you're not going to use the lumen immediately, heparinize the catheter.

• If you can't get blood flowing from the catheter, the tip of the catheter could be against the vessel wall. To correct this, ask the patient to raise his arms over his head, turn on his side, cough, or perform the Valsalva maneuver. You can also try flushing the catheter with saline solution before making another attempt to draw blood.

If evacuated tubes aren't available, obtain the blood sample with a syringe (see *Drawing blood with a syringe,* page 94).

Documenting the infusion. Record your assessment findings and interventions according to your hospital's policy. Include the following information:
• the type, amount, and rate of infusion
• dressing changes, including the appearance and location of the catheter and the site, as well as how the patient tolerated the procedure
• tubing and solution changes
• cap changes
• flushings, including any problems encountered, and the amount and type of solution used
• other solutions infused
• blood samples collected, including the type and amount.

Correcting common problems
Besides performing routine care measures, you must be prepared to handle common problems that may arise during infusion. For instance, you may need to repair a torn catheter or replace a dislodged or disconnected one.

Maintaining CV therapy also involves preventing catheter kinks by taping and positioning the catheter properly. For example, looping the tubing once and securing it with tape on top of the dressing prevents the catheter from being pulled if

Drawing blood with a syringe

Before obtaining a blood sample from your patient's central venous catheter, you'll need to collect the following equipment: syringes, evacuated tubes for the sample, gloves, and saline or heparin flush solution.

After you've gathered the equipment, draw the blood using these steps:
• Stop all infusions.
• Select the port you'll be using to withdraw the blood; it should be at least 20G – preferably 16G or 18G.
• Put on gloves.
• Using aseptic technique, disconnect the tubing or heparin lock cap. (If the catheter has a clamp, use it before disconnecting; if the catheter doesn't have a clamp, have the patient perform the Valsalva maneuver.)
• Insert the syringe and draw back 5 ml of blood.
• Discard the syringe.
• Connect a second syringe and draw the amount of blood you need.
• Flush the catheter with the recommended amount of saline solution or heparin. (The amount depends on the type of catheter and the frequency and type of infusions. Check the manufacturer's recommendations and your hospital's policy.)
• Place the blood in the evacuated tubes.
• Label the evacuated tubes and send them to the laboratory.

the tubing gets caught on something. This technique also helps prevent the catheter from moving at the insertion site – a major cause of catheter-related infections.

Finally, you need to know how to manage clot formation at the lumen tip, a potentially serious problem that can impede the infusion, make blood samples more difficult to obtain, and lead to infection. (See

Managing common problems.)

Repairing or replacing a catheter. A serrated hemostat will eventually break down the silicone rubber and tear the catheter, causing blood to back up and fluid to leak from the site. If air enters the catheter through the tear, an embolism may result. You can prevent catheter tears by using nonserrated clamps. You may also be able to repair a torn long-term catheter. (See *Repairing a long-term CV catheter,* page 97.)

Some hospitals permit nurses to make temporary repairs on short-term multilumen catheters, using the same technique you would use on a long-term catheter. For example, you might repair a short-term catheter to keep a lumen patent when one of its extensions breaks. Generally, however, the doctor will replace it with a new one as soon as possible.

Unkinking a twisted catheter. The catheter can kink either above or beneath the skin. Kinks beneath the skin are detected by an X-ray and can sometimes be corrected by repositioning the patient. If repositioning doesn't remove the kink, the catheter must be replaced.

Never attempt to straighten kinks in stiff catheters, such as those made from PVC; these catheters fracture easily, and fractured particles may enter the circulation. The doctor may try to unkink a long-term catheter because it's made of pliable silicone rubber.

Managing clot formation. Difficulty withdrawing blood or infusing fluid may be due to clot formation at the tip of the catheter. A clot not only impedes the flow of blood and fluid but also provides a protein-rich

Managing common problems

Maintaining central venous therapy means being prepared to handle problems that may arise. The following chart tells you how to recognize and manage some common problems.

PROBLEM	POSSIBLE CAUSES	NURSING INTERVENTIONS
Fluid won't infuse	• Closed clamp • Displaced or kinked catheter • Thrombus	• Check the infusion system and clamps. • Change the patient's position. • Have the patient cough, breathe deeply, or perform the Valsalva maneuver. • Remove dressing and examine external portion of catheter. • If a kink isn't apparent, obtain an X-ray order. • Try to withdraw blood. • Try a gentle flush with saline solution. (The doctor may order a thrombolytic flush.)
Unable to draw blood	• Closed clamp • Displaced or kinked catheter • Thrombus • Catheter movement against vessel wall with negative pressure	• Check the infusion system and clamps. • Change the patient's position. • Have the patient cough, breathe deeply, or perform the Valsalva maneuver. • Remove dressing and examine external portion of catheter. • Obtain an X-ray order.
Fluid leaking at the site	• Displaced catheter • Lymph fluid leaking from subcutaneous tract • Tear in catheter	• Check patient for signs of distress. • Change dressing and observe site for redness. • Notify the doctor. • Obtain an X-ray order. • Prepare for a catheter change, if necessary. • If tear occurred in a Hickman, Groshong, or Broviac catheter, obtain a repair kit.
Disconnected catheter	• Patient movement • Not securely connected to tubing	• Apply catheter clamp, if available. • Place sterile syringe or catheter plug in the catheter hub. • Change the I.V. extension set. *Don't* reconnect the contaminated tubing. • Clean the catheter hub with alcohol or povidone-iodine. Don't soak the hub. • Connect clean I.V. tubing or a heparin lock plug to the site. • Restart the infusion. *(continued)*

Managing common problems (continued)

PROBLEM	POSSIBLE CAUSES	NURSING INTERVENTIONS
Obstructed catheter	• Thrombus • Improper flushing • Decreased flow rate • Precipitate formation from infusion of incompatible substances • Catheter improperly positioned in vein; catheter tip against vessel wall	• Reposition patient and check for flow. • Attempt to aspirate the clot. Don't force clot. • Notify the doctor. • Possibly, infuse thrombolytic agents such as streptokinase or urokinase. • Possibly, remove catheter (may be repositioned in vein with verification by X-ray). • Document interventions.

environment for bacterial growth.

Occasionally, the clot forms in such a way that fluids infuse easily, while blood aspiration is difficult or impossible. The fibrin clot may be dissolved by administering urokinase, a thrombolytic agent (5,000 units in 3 ml of saline solution). Usually performed by a doctor, this procedure is recommended for long-term CV catheters because they're difficult and costly to replace.

Patients with special needs
You'll need to tailor certain aspects of your nursing care if you have either a pediatric, elderly, or home-therapy patient. For instance, a patient who will be receiving CV home therapy will need considerably more teaching to ensure both his safety and the success of his treatment.

Pediatric and elderly patients. Although the same catheters are used in both pediatric and elderly patients, the length and lumen size may differ, as may the insertion sites. In infants, for example, the jugular vein is the preferred insertion site, even though it's much more difficult to maintain than other sites. Usually, the doctor and the patient's family will select a mutually acceptable site if the catheter will be used for long-term therapy. The amount of fluid infused in a pediatric patient will, of course, also vary depending upon the size of the patient.

Home-therapy patients. Long-term CV catheters allow patients to receive caustic fluids and blood infusions at home. These catheters have a much longer life because they are less thrombogenic and less prone to infection than short-term devices.

A candidate for home therapy must have a family member or friend who can safely and competently administer the I.V. fluids, a backup helper, a suitable home environment, a telephone, transportation, adequate reading skills, and the ability to prepare, handle, store, and dispose of the equipment. The care procedures used in the home are the same as those used in the hospital, except the home-therapy patient uses clean technique instead of aseptic technique.

The overall goal of home therapy is patient safety, so your patient teaching must begin well before discharge. After discharge, a home-therapy coordinator will provide follow-up care until the patient or someone close to him can independently provide catheter care and infusion therapy. Many home-therapy patients learn to care for the catheter themselves and to infuse their own medications and solutions.

Complications of CV therapy

Complications can occur any time during the infusion therapy. Traumatic complications, such as pneumothorax, typically occur upon insertion but may not be noticed until after the procedure is completed. Systemic complications, such as sepsis, typically occur later during the infusion.

Traumatic complications. The most common traumatic complication, pneumothorax is associated with insertions of subclavian or internal jugular lines. It's usually discovered in the chest X-ray that confirms catheter placement.

Unless the patient is on positive-pressure ventilation, the pneumothorax is usually minimal and may not require intervention. If the pneumothorax is large enough to cause such signs and symptoms as chest pain, dyspnea, cyanosis, or decreased or absent breath sounds on the affected side, a thoracotomy should be performed and a chest tube inserted.

Initially, the patient may be asymptomatic but will gradually show signs of distress as the pneumothorax gets larger. For this reason, you need to monitor the patient closely and auscultate breath

Repairing a long-term CV catheter

When a patient's long-term central venous (CV) catheter is torn or damaged, you may be able to repair it. Some long-term catheters have prepackaged permanent repair kits. If such a kit isn't available, you can make a temporary repair by following these steps:
• Immediately clamp the catheter between the chest wall and the tear.
• Clean the torn area with povidone-iodine.
• Using sterile scissors, cut off the damaged portion, as shown.

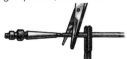

• Insert a blunt-end needle with the appropriate gauge (usually a 14G or 16G) into the distal end of the catheter, as shown.

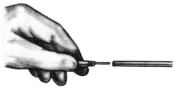

• Place an injection cap in the hub of the needle as shown and heparinize the catheter.

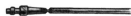

• Tie a silk suture around the needle and catheter to secure them.
• Release the clamp.
• Check the repaired catheter for leaks by flushing it with saline solution.
• Tell the doctor you've made an emergency repair; when possible, he may want it redone with a permanent repair kit—a procedure that involves splicing a new section of catheter with an end connector to the rest of the catheter.

sounds for at least 8 hours after catheter insertion.

If unchecked, pneumothorax may progress to tension pneumothorax, a medical emergency. The patient will exhibit signs of acute respiratory distress, asymmetrical chest wall movement, and possibly a tracheal shift away from the affected side. A chest tube must be inserted immediately before respiratory and cardiac decompensation occur.

The second most common traumatic complication, arterial puncture may lead to hemothorax or internal bleeding, which may not be detected immediately. A hemothorax is treated in the same manner as a pneumothorax, except that the chest tube is inserted lower in the chest

If untreated, internal bleeding caused by arterial puncture will lead to hypovolemic shock. Signs and symptoms include increased heart rate; decreased blood pressure; cool, clammy skin; obvious swelling in the neck or chest; mental confusion (especially if the common carotid arteries are involved); and hematoma formation, which causes pressure on the trachea and adjacent vessels.

A relatively rare complication, tracheal puncture is associated with insertions of subclavian lines. Also rare, fistula development between the innominate vein and the subclavian artery results from perforation with the guidewire upon insertion of a subclavian venous catheter.

Systemic complications. Of these complications, catheter-related sepsis is the most serious. It may lead to septic shock, multisystem organ failure, and death. Most sepsis attributed to CV catheters is caused by skin surface organisms, such as *Staphylococcus epidermidis, S.*

aureus, and *Candida albicans.*

Strict aseptic technique and close observation are the best defenses against sepsis. Regularly check the catheter insertion site for signs of localized infection, such as tenderness along the catheter path. If the patient shows signs of generalized infection, such as unexplained fever, draw blood cultures from a peripheral site as well as the catheter itself.

If catheter-related sepsis is suspected, the catheter may be removed and a new one inserted in a different site. Culture the catheter tip after removal. Administer antibiotics, as ordered, and draw repeat blood cultures after the antibiotic course is complete.

Other common complications associated with CV therapy include phlebitis (especially in peripheral CV therapy) and thrombus formation. (See *Risks of CV therapy.*)

Discontinuing CV therapy

The task of discontinuing CV therapy and removing the catheter may be yours or the doctor's, depending on the hospital's policy and the type of catheter. For instance, long-term catheters and implantable devices are always removed by the doctor, usually under surgical conditions. But PICC lines may be removed by a qualified nurse.

You may receive an order to discontinue continuous infusion therapy and begin intermittent infusion therapy. If so, follow the same procedure used for peripheral I.V. therapy.

Removing the catheter. If you're qualified to remove the catheter, first check the patient's record for the most recent placement confirmed by an X-ray to trace the

(Text continues on page 102.)

COMPLICATIONS

Risks of CV therapy

As with any invasive procedure, central venous (CV) therapy poses risks, including pneumothorax, air embolism, thrombosis, and infection. The following chart outlines how to prevent these common complications—and how to recognize and manage them when they occur.

SIGNS AND SYMPTOMS	POSSIBLE CAUSES	NURSING INTERVENTIONS
Pneumothorax, hemothorax, chylothorax, or hydrothorax		
• Chest pain • Dyspnea • Cyanosis • Decreased breath sounds on affected side • With hemothorax, decreased hemoglobin because of blood pooling • Abnormal chest X-ray	• Lung puncture by catheter during insertion or exchange over a guidewire • Large blood vessel puncture with bleeding inside or outside of lung • Lymph node puncture with leakage of lymph fluid • Infusion of solution into chest area through infiltrated catheter	• Notify doctor. • Remove catheter or assist with removal. • Administer oxygen as ordered. • Set up and assist with chest tube insertion. • Document interventions. *Prevention:* • Position patient's head down with a towel roll between the scapulae to dilate and expose the internal jugular or subclavian vein as much as possible during catheter insertion. • Assess for early signs of fluid infiltration, such as swelling in shoulder, neck, chest, and arm area. • Ensure immobilization of patient with adequate preparation for procedure and restraint during procedure; active patients may need to be sedated or taken to the operating room for CV catheter insertion. • Minimize patient activity after insertion, especially if peripheral CV catheter is used.
Air embolism		
• Respiratory distress • Unequal breath sounds • Weak pulse • Increased central venous pressure (CVP) • Decreased blood pressure • Churning murmur over precordium	• Intake of air into CV system during catheter insertion, tubing changes; inadvertent opening, cutting, or breaking of catheter	• Clamp catheter immediately. • Turn patient on his left side, head down, so air can enter right atrium and be dispersed via pulmonary artery. Maintain position for 20 to 30 minutes. • Don't have the patient perform the Valsalva maneuver. (A large intake of air would worsen the situation.) • Administer oxygen. • Notify doctor. • Document interventions.

(continued)

COMPLICATIONS

 Risks of CV therapy *(continued)*

SIGNS AND SYMPTOMS	POSSIBLE CAUSES	NURSING INTERVENTIONS
Air embolism *(continued)*		
• Change in or loss of consciousness		*Prevention:* • Purge all air from tubing before hookup. • Teach patient to perform the Valsalva maneuver during catheter insertion and tubing changes (bear down or strain and hold breath to increase CVP). • Use air-eliminating filters proximal to patient. • Use infusion-control device with air detection capability. • Use luer-lock tubing, tape connections, or use locking devices for all connections.
Thrombosis		
• Edema at puncture site • Erythema • Ipsilateral swelling of arm, neck, and face • Pain along vein • Fever, malaise • Tachycardia	• Sluggish flow rate • Composition of catheter material (some materials such as polyvinyl-chloride are more thrombogenic) • Hematopoietic status of patient • Preexisting limb edema • Infusion of irritating solutions • Repeated use of same vein or long-term use • Preexisting cardiovascular disease	• Notify doctor. • Possibly, remove catheter. • Possibly, infuse anticoagulant doses of heparin. • Verify thrombosis with diagnostic studies. • Apply warm wet compresses locally. • Don't use limb on affected side for subsequent venipuncture. • Document interventions. *Prevention:* • Maintain flow through catheter at steady rate with infusion pump, or flush at regular intervals. • Use catheters made of less thrombogenic materials or catheters coated to prevent thrombosis. • Dilute irritating solutions. • Use 0.22-micron filter for infusions.
Local infection		
• Redness, warmth, tenderness, swelling at insertion or exit site • Possible exudate of purulent material • Local rash or pustules • Fever, chills, malaise	• Failure to maintain aseptic technique during catheter insertion or care • Failure to comply with dressing change protocol • Wet or soiled dressing remaining on site	• Monitor temperature frequently. • Culture site. • Redress aseptically. • Possibly, use antibiotic ointment locally. • Treat systemically with antibiotics or antifungals, depending on culture results and doctor's order. • Catheter may be removed. • Document interventions.

Risks of CV therapy (continued)

SIGNS AND SYMPTOMS	POSSIBLE CAUSES	NURSING INTERVENTIONS
Local infection (continued)		
	• Immunosuppression • Irritated suture line	*Prevention:* • Maintain strict aseptic technique. Use gloves, masks, and gowns when appropriate. • Adhere to dressing change protocols. • Teach patient about restrictions on swimming, bathing, and so on. (Patients with adequate white blood cell counts can do these activities if doctor allows.) • Change wet or soiled dressing immediately. • Change dressing more frequently if catheter is located in femoral area or near tracheostomy. Complete trach care after catheter care.
Systemic infection		
• Fever, chills without other apparent reason • Leukocytosis • Nausea, vomiting • Malaise • Elevated urine glucose level	• Contaminated catheter or infusate • Failure to maintain aseptic technique during solution hookup • Frequent opening of catheter or long-term use of single I.V. access • Immunosuppression	• Draw central and peripheral blood cultures; if same organism, catheter is primary source of sepsis and should be removed. • If cultures don't match but are positive, catheter may be removed or the infection may be treated through the catheter. • Treat patient with antibiotic regimen, as ordered. • Culture tip of catheter if removed. • Assess for other sources of infection. • Monitor vital signs closely. • Document interventions. *Prevention:* • Examine infusate for cloudiness and turbidity before infusing, and check fluid container for leaks. • Monitor urine glucose level in total parenteral nutrition patients; if greater than 2+, suspect early sepsis. • Use strict sterile technique for hookup and disconnection of fluids. • Use 0.22-micron filter. • Catheter may be changed frequently to decrease chance of infection. • Keep the system closed as much as possible. • Teach patient aseptic technique.

catheter's path as it exits the body. Make sure that backup assistance is available if a complication, such as uncontrolled bleeding, occurs during catheter removal. (Some vessels, such as the subclavian vein, are difficult to compress.) Before you remove the catheter, explain the procedure to the patient. Tell him that he'll need to perform the Valsalva maneuver when the catheter is withdrawn. If necessary, review the maneuver with him.

Before removing the catheter, gather this equipment: sterile gauze, hemostat, clean gloves, sterile gloves, forceps, sterile scissors, povidone-iodine solution, alcohol swabs, a transparent semipermeable dressing, and tape. If the tip of the catheter will be sent for culture, you'll also need a sterile specimen container and an extra pair of sterile scissors.

Now, follow these steps:
• Place the patient in a supine position to prevent emboli.
• Wash your hands and put on clean gloves.
• Turn off all infusions and prepare a sterile field.
• Remove the old dressing and change to sterile gloves.
• Prep the site first with alcohol, then with povidone-iodine solution. Inspect the site for signs of drainage or inflammation.
• Clip the sutures and remove the catheter in a slow, even motion. Have the patient perform the Valsalva maneuver as the catheter is withdrawn to prevent air emboli.
• Apply povidone-iodine ointment to the insertion site to seal it.
• Inspect the catheter to see if any portions broke off during the removal. If so, notify the doctor immediately and monitor the patient closely for signs of distress. If a culture is to be obtained, clip ap-

proximately 1" (2.5 cm) off the distal end of the catheter, letting it drop into the sterile specimen container.
• Place a transparent semipermeable dressing over the site. Label the dressing with the date and time of the removal and your initials.
• Properly dispose of the I.V. tubing and equipment you used.

Document the time and date of the catheter removal, and any complications that occurred, such as catheter shearing, bleeding, or respiratory distress. Also be sure to record signs of blood, drainage, redness, or swelling of the site.

Make a notation on the nursing care plan to recheck the patient and insertion site frequently for the next few hours. Check for signs of respiratory decompensation, possibly indicating air emboli, and for signs of bleeding, such as blood on the dressing, decreased blood pressure, increased heart rate, paleness, or diaphoresis.

Remember that some vessels aren't easily compressed and that insidious bleeding may develop after removing the catheter. By 72 hours, the site should be sealed and the risk of air emboli should be past; however, you may still need to apply a dry dressing to the site.

Suggested readings

Damen, J., and Van der Tweel, I. "Positive Tip Cultures and Related Risk Factors Associated with Intravascular Catheterization in Pediatric Cardiac Patients," *Critical Care Medicine* 16(3):221-28, March 1988.

Darovic, G. *Hemodynamic Monitoring: Invasive and Noninvasive Clinical Applications.* Philadelphia: W.B. Saunders Co., 1987.

Harvey, W.H., et al. "A Prospective

Evaluation of the Port-A-Cath Implantable Venous Access System in Chronically Ill Adults and Children,'' *Surgery, Gynecology and Obstetrics* 169(6):495-500, December 1989.

Johansen, B., et al. *Standards for Critical Care,* 3rd ed. St. Louis: C.V. Mosby Co., 1988.

Kozier, B., and Erb, G. *Techniques in Clinical Nursing,* 3rd ed. Reading, Mass.: Addison-Wesley Publishing Co., 1989.

Luckmann, J., and Sorensen, K.C. *Medical Surgical Nursing,* 3rd ed. Philadelphia: W.B. Saunders Co., 1987.

Pabst, T., et al. ''Subclavian Artery-to-Innominate Vein Fistula: A Case Caused By Subclavian Venous Catheterization,'' *Surgery* 105(6):801-03, June 1989.

Plumer, A. *Principles and Practices of Intravenous Therapy,* 4th ed. Boston: Little, Brown & Co., 1987.

Sohl, L., and Nze, R. ''Working with Triple Lumen Central Venous Catheters,'' *Nursing88* 18(7):50-55, July 1988.

Sundberg, M. *Fundamentals of Nursing with Clinical Procedures,* 2nd ed. Boston: Jones and Bartlett Publishers, 1989.

Textbook of Advanced Cardiac Life Support. Dallas: American Heart Association, 1987.

Tucker, S., et al. *Patient Care Standards,* 4th ed. St. Louis: C.V. Mosby Co., 1988.

Underhill, S., et al. *Cardiac Nursing,* 2nd ed. Philadelphia: J.B. Lippincott Co., 1989.

Viall, C. ''Your Complete Guide to Central Venous Catheters,'' *Nursing90* 20(2):34-42, February 1990.

4

THERAPY WITH IMPLANTED VASCULAR ACCESS DEVICES

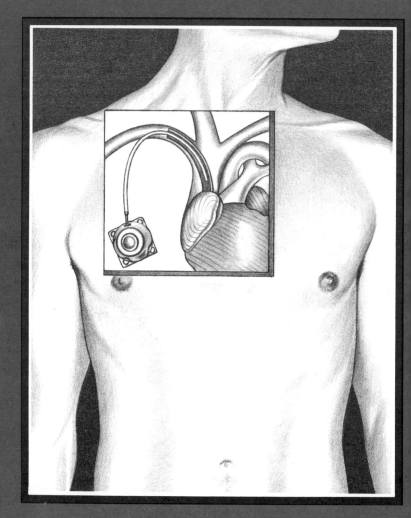

As the number of chronically ill patients increases, so does the need for long-term I.V. therapy. And that means you'll be caring for more and more patients who have implanted vascular access devices.

Typically, an implantable device will be selected when an external catheter isn't desirable for a patient who needs long-term I.V. access. To care for such a patient before and after the device is implanted, you must understand some basic principles and procedures.

This chapter explains how the most common type of vascular access device—the vascular access port (VAP)—works and spells out the techniques for administering, maintaining, and discontinuing infusion therapy. The chapter also discusses routine nursing care, including how to manage common problems and potential complications of the vascular access device.

Basics of therapy

Implanted in a pocket under the skin, a VAP functions much like a long-term central venous (CV) catheter, except that it has no external parts. (See *Comparing VAPs and long-term CV catheters*, page 106.) The attached indwelling catheter tunnels through the subcutaneous tissue so the catheter tip lies in a central vein—the subclavian vein, for example. A VAP can also be used for arterial access or implanted into the epidural space, peritoneum, or pericardial or pleural cavity.

Typically, VAPs deliver intermittent infusions. Most often used for chemotherapy, a VAP can also deliver I.V. fluids, medications, or blood products. Plus, you can use a VAP to obtain blood samples.

Traditionally, VAPs haven't been used to deliver total parenteral nutrition (TPN) because the daily needle punctures needed to access the port could lead to skin breakdown. Similarly, VAPs haven't been used for long-term antibiotic therapy because of the need for almost continuous access to the port. The devices should be used with caution in patients unable to tolerate other implantable devices and those with a high risk of developing an allergic reaction or infection.

Advantages and disadvantages

VAPs offer several advantages, including minimal activity restrictions, few self-care measures for the patient to learn and perform, and few dressing changes (except when used to maintain continuous infusions or heparin locks). Implanted devices are easier to maintain than external devices. For instance, they require heparinization only once after each use (or periodically, when not in use). They also pose less risk of infection because they have no exit site to serve as an entry for microorganisms.

Finally, because VAPs create only a slight protrusion under the skin, many patients find them easier to accept than external infusion devices. A patient with a VAP can shower, swim, and exercise without worrying about the device.

Because the device is implanted, however, it may be more difficult for the patient to manage, particularly if he'll be administering medications or fluids on a daily or frequent basis. And since accessing the device requires inserting a needle through subcutaneous tissue, patients who fear or dislike needle punctures may be uncomfortable

Comparing VAPs and long-term CV catheters

A vascular access port (VAP) offers patients many of the advantages of a long-term central venous (CV) catheter, along with an unobtrusive design that many patients find easier to accept. Both devices are indicated when poor venous access prohibits peripheral I.V. therapy. Deciding which device to use depends on the type and duration of treatment, the frequency of access, and the patient's criteria. The following chart shows how the two devices compare.

CRITERIA	VAP	LONG-TERM CV CATHETER
Type of treatment		
Continuous infusion of drugs or fluids	Yes, but maintaining continuous needle access eliminates the benefits of implantation	Yes
Self-administration of drugs or fluids	Yes, but may be more difficult for patient or family member to manage	Yes
Bolus injections of vesicant or irritant drugs by health care professionals	Yes	Yes
Duration of treatment		
Less than 3 months	No, due to the high cost of implanting and removing the device	Yes
More than 3 months	Yes, but cost of implantation and removal may preclude cost benefit if treatment lasts less than 6 months	Yes
Frequency of access		
Three or more times a week	Yes, but may minimize the advantage of having an implanted device	Yes
Less than once a week	Yes	No, due to the high cost of maintaining the catheter
Patient concerns		
Negative effect on body image	No	Possibly
Negative reaction to needle punctures	Possibly	No
Ability to care for external catheter needed	No	Yes
Cost of dressing changes and heparinization	Minimal	Considerable

using it. In addition, the implantation and removal of the implantable device requires surgery and hospitalization, which can be costly. The comparatively high cost of VAPs makes them worthwhile only for patients who require infusion therapy for at least 6 months. (See *A close-up look at a VAP*. Also, for information on another type of implantable vascular access device, see *Understanding implantable pumps,* page 108.)

Preparing for implantation and infusion

Before the VAP is implanted, you need to prepare the patient for the procedure. Preparation for therapy also includes selecting the type of VAP and the implantation site. Typically, the doctor will make these choices.

Preparing the patient

Before therapy begins, make sure the patient understands the procedure, its benefit to him, and what's expected of him during and after the implantation. Although the primary responsibility for explaining the procedure and its goals rests with the doctor, you must be prepared to supplement his explanation. You'll also need to allay the patient's fears and answer questions about movement restrictions, cosmetic concerns, and management regimens. Your ability to explain the procedure and the patient's role helps ensure his cooperation and the therapy's success.

Explaining the procedure. Ask your patient if he's ever received an

EQUIPMENT

A close-up look at a VAP

A vascular access port (VAP) consists of a catheter connected to a small reservoir. A septum designed to withstand multiple punctures seals the reservoir.

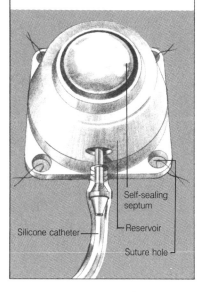

Silicone catheter

Self-sealing septum

Reservoir

Suture hole

I.V. infusion or had an implanted device. Evaluate his learning capabilities, and adjust your teaching technique accordingly. For example, use age-appropriate language to describe the procedure to a child. If available, use pictures and physical models to help the patient understand.

To encourage the patient's cooperation, explain the entire implantation procedure. Be sure to describe how he'll be positioned during the procedure. If it'll be performed under general anesthesia—a rare occurrence—emphasize preoperative and postoperative care measures.

Also explain any diagnostic tests

EQUIPMENT

Understanding implantable pumps

Usually placed in a subcutaneous pocket made in the abdomen below the umbilicus, an implantable pump has two chambers separated by a bellows. One chamber contains the I.V. solution, while the other contains a charging fluid. The charging fluid chamber exerts continuous pressure on the bellows, forcing the infusion solution through the silicone outlet catheter into a central vein. The pump also has an auxiliary septum that can be used to deliver bolus injections of medication. Generally, the pump is indicated for patients who require continuous low-volume infusions.

TOP VIEW

CROSS-SECTIONAL VIEW

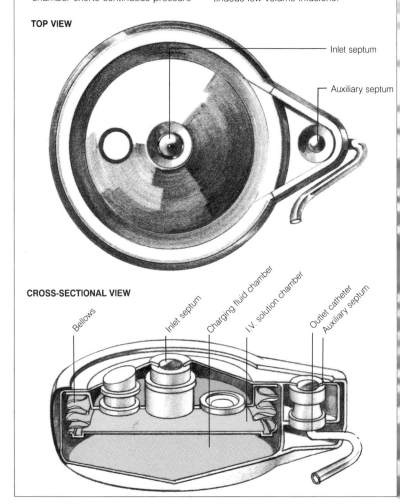

hat may be done. Some doctors order a venogram before implantation to determine the best vessel to use. After the procedure, a chest X-ray or fluoroscopy confirms placement of the device. Also, blood samples may be drawn to establish baseline coagulation profiles.

Explaining postoperative care. Tell the patient that once the device is in place, he'll have to keep scheduled appointments to have the port heparinized. Also, teach him to report signs and symptoms of systemic infection (fever, malaise, and flulike symptoms) and local infection (redness, tenderness, and drainage at the port or tunnel track site). Explain that he'll need to receive prophylactic antibiotics before undergoing any dental or surgical procedures, and tell him to inform his dentist or doctor that he's using an implanted device.

Teach the patient to recognize and report signs and symptoms of infiltration, such as pain or swelling at the site, especially if he'll be receiving continuous infusions. Stress the need for immediate intervention to avoid damaging the tissue surrounding the port.

Obtaining consent. Most hospitals require an informed consent before any invasive procedure. The doctor will obtain the consent and, in most cases, you'll be responsible for witnessing the patient's signature. Tell the patient he'll be asked to sign a consent form and explain what this means. Before he signs, make sure he understands the procedure.

In the case of a rare emergency implantation, the consent form may be signed by the next of kin, or administrative approval may be granted. However, you should still teach the patient about his therapy — even if the teaching occurs after the device is implanted.

Selecting the equipment

The VAP selected for a patient depends on the type of therapy he needs and how often he needs access to the port. Typically, VAPs are used for intermittent infusions and only require access during therapy.

The VAP and its implantation site, in turn, affect the selection of the infusion equipment. Generally, the equipment is the same as that used in peripheral I.V. and CV therapy and includes the infusion solution and an administration set with tubing.

Choosing the VAP. A VAP consists of a silicone catheter attached to a reservoir, which is covered with a self-sealing silicone rubber septum. One- and two-piece units with single or double lumens are available.

VAPs come in two basic types: top entry and side entry. In a top-entry VAP (such as the Med-i-Port, Port-A-Cath, and Infuse-A-Port), the needle is inserted perpendicular to the reservoir. In a side-entry VAP (such as the S.E.A. Port), the needle is inserted almost parallel to the reservoir. (See *Comparing top-entry and side-entry VAPs,* page 110.)

The VAP reservoir can be made of titanium, such as the Port-A-Cath; stainless steel, such as the Q-Port; or molded plastic, such as the Infuse-A-Port. The type selected depends on the patient's therapeutic needs. For example, a cancer patient undergoing magnetic resonance imaging (MRI) should use a device made of titanium or plastic instead of stainless steel to avoid distorting the MRI image.

The VAP catheter comes with one

EQUIPMENT

Comparing top-entry and side-entry VAPs

Vascular access ports (VAPs) come in two basic designs: top entry and side entry. In a top-entry port, the needle is inserted perpendicular to the reservoir. In a side-entry port, the needle is inserted into the septum nearly parallel to the reservoir. (A needle stop prevents the needle from coming out of the other side of the port.)

TOP-ENTRY VAP

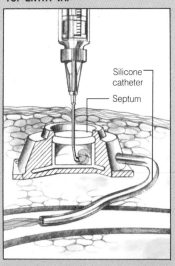

Silicone catheter

Septum

SIDE-ENTRY VAP

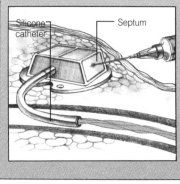

Silicone catheter

Septum

or two large or small lumens, depending on the patient's size and the type of therapy. For example, blood sampling or transfusion therapy requires a larger-size lumen than does I.V. fluid administration.

Choosing the VAP needle. To avoid damaging the port's silicone rubber septum, you should use only non-coring needles with a VAP. A non-coring needle has an angled or deflected point that slices the septum upon entry, rather than coring it as a conventional needle will do. When the non-coring needle is removed, the septum will then reseal itself. (See *Identifying non-coring needles.*)

Non-coring needles come with metal or plastic hubs in straight or right-angle configurations, with or without an extension set. Each configuration comes in various lengths (depending on the depth of septum implantation) and gauges (depending on the type and rate of the infusion). For example, experts recommend using a 19G needle for blood infusion or withdrawal; a 20G needle for most other infusions, including TPN; and a 22G needle for flushing. Most often, you'll use a right-angle non-coring needle; rarely, you'll need a longer needle, such as a straight 2″ non-coring needle, to access a deeply implanted port.

You can use either a straight needle or a right-angle needle to inject a bolus into a top-entry port. For continuous infusions, however, experts recommend using a right-angle needle because it's easily secured to the patient. Side-entry ports are designed exclusively for use with straight non-coring needles.

• *Over-the-needle catheters.* An over-the-needle catheter, such as

EQUIPMENT

Identifying non-coring needles

Unlike a conventional hypodermic needle, a non-coring needle has a deflected point, which slices the port's septum instead of coring it. Non-coring needles come in two types: straight and right angle.

Generally, expect to use a right-angle needle with a top-entry port, and a straight needle with a side-entry port. When administering a bolus injection or continuous infusion, you'll also use an extension set.

Conventional hypodermic needle

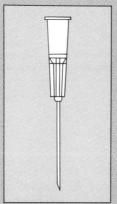

Straight non-coring needle

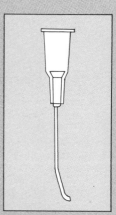

Right-angle non-coring needle

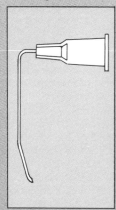

Right-angle non-coring needle with extension set

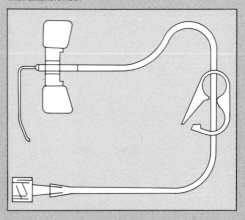

the Surecath device, can give you continuous access to the port. This style catheter has the benefit of offering the patient greater comfort with less risk the device will migrate out of the septum. A solid-spike introducer and flexible cathe-ter are passed through the silicone septum; then the introducer is re-moved, and the flexible Teflon cath-eter is positioned to the contour of the patient's chest wall. (See *Using an over-the-needle catheter,* page 112.)

EQUIPMENT

Using an over-the-needle catheter

An over-the-needle catheter, such as the Surecath device shown below, provides continuous access to an implanted port. The Surecath consists of a solid-spike introducer and a flexible catheter, which you pass through the portal septum and into the chamber. You then withdraw the introducer, leaving the catheter in place.

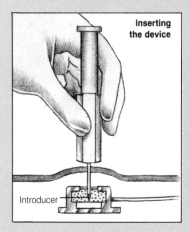

Inserting the device

Introducer

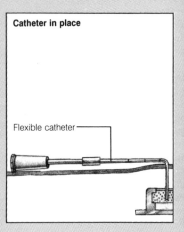

Catheter in place

Flexible catheter

Assisting with implantation and initiating therapy

Before therapy can begin, a doctor needs to surgically implant the VAP. In most cases, he'll do this using local anesthesia, although sometimes he may use general anesthesia.

Implanting the device
First the doctor makes a small incision and introduces the catheter into the superior vena cava through either the subclavian, jugular, or cephalic vein. After fluoroscopy verifies placement of the catheter

tip, he creates a subcutaneous pocket over a bony prominence in the chest wall. He then tunnels the catheter to the pocket.

Next, he connects the catheter to the reservoir, places the reservoir in the pocket, and flushes it with heparin solution. Then he sutures the reservoir to the underlying fascia and closes the incision.

During the implantation procedure, you may be responsible for handing equipment and supplies to the doctor, as you would for a CV catheter insertion.

Monitoring the patient
After the VAP is implanted, observe the patient for several hours. The device can be used immediately after placement, although some

edema and tenderness may persist for about 72 hours. This makes the device initially difficult to palpate and slightly uncomfortable for the patient.

The incision requires routine postoperative care for 7 to 10 days. You'll also need to assess the implantation site for signs of infection, hematoma, device rotation, or skin erosion. You don't need to apply a dressing to the wound site, except during infusions or to maintain a heparin lock.

Initiating therapy

After the doctor has implanted the device, you'll need to set up the equipment and prepare the site so you can initiate therapy. Then you can access the port, following the specific steps for top-entry or side-entry ports, and administer a bolus injection or initiate a continuous infusion, as ordered.

Setting up the equipment. Attach the tubing to the solution container, prime the tubing with fluid, fill the syringes with saline or heparin flush solution, and prime the non-coring needle and extension set. All priming must be done using strict aseptic technique, and all tubing must be free of air. After you've primed the tubing, recheck all the connections for tightness. Make sure that all open ends are covered with sealed caps.

Preparing the site. After you've set up the equipment, prepare the insertion site. First, obtain an implantable port access kit, if your hospital uses them. If one of these kits isn't available, gather the equipment you'll need: sterile gloves, three alcohol swabs, three povidone-iodine swabs, an ice pack, and a local anesthetic (optional).

Then, using aseptic technique, follow these steps:
• Inspect the area around the port for signs of infection or skin breakdown.
• Place an ice pack over the area for several minutes to alleviate possible discomfort of the needle puncture.
• Wash your hands thoroughly and put on sterile gloves. Remember to keep these gloves on throughout the procedure.
• Clean the area with an alcohol swab, starting at the center of the port and working outward with a firm circular motion over a 4″ to 5″ (10.2 to 12.7 cm) diameter. Repeat this procedure twice.
• Clean the area with a povidone-iodine swab in the same manner described above. Repeat this procedure twice.
• If hospital policy calls for a local anesthetic, check the patient's record for possible allergies. As indicated, anesthetize the insertion site by injecting 0.1 ml of xylocaine (without adrenaline).

Accessing a top-entry port. After the site is prepared, gather the equipment you'll need: usually a right-angle non-coring needle and a 5-ml syringe filled with saline solution. Then follow these steps:
• Palpate the area over the port to locate the port septum.
• Anchor the port between your thumb and the first two fingers of your nondominant hand. Then using your dominant hand, aim the needle at the center of the device.
• Insert the needle perpendicular to the port septum. Push the needle through the skin and septum until you reach the bottom of the reservoir. (See *Securing a top-entry VAP,* page 114.)
• Check needle placement by aspirating for a blood return.

Securing a top-entry VAP

This illustration shows the correct way to secure a top-entry vascular access port (VAP). Hold the device between your thumb and first two fingers while inserting a needle into the septum.

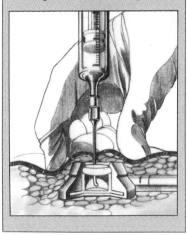

• If you're unable to obtain blood, remove the needle and repeat the procedure. Inability to obtain blood might indicate that the catheter is against the vessel's wall. Ask the patient to raise his arms, perform the Valsalva maneuver, or change position in order to free the catheter. If you still can't obtain a blood return, notify the doctor: A fibrin sleeve on the distal end of the catheter may be occluding the opening.
• Flush the device with saline solution. If you detect swelling or if the patient reports pain at the site, remove the needle and notify the doctor.

Accessing a side-entry port. To gain access to a side-entry port, you'll follow the same basic procedure you'd use to access a top-entry port. However, you'll insert the needle parallel to the reservoir, instead of perpendicular to it.

While the patient is hospitalized, a luer-lock injection cap may be attached to the end of the extension set to provide ready access for intermittent infusions. Besides saving valuable nursing time, a luer-lock will reduce the discomfort of accessing the port, as well as prolong the life of the port septum by decreasing the number of needle punctures.

Administering a bolus injection.
After you've accessed the port, you can administer a bolus injection, as ordered. First gather the following equipment: an extension set, a clamp, a 10-ml syringe filled with saline solution, a syringe containing the prescribed medication, and a sterile needle filled with heparin flush solution (optional). Then follow these steps:
• Attach the 10-ml syringe filled with saline solution to the end of the extension set and remove all the air. Now attach the extension set to the non-coring needle.
• Check for a blood return. Then flush the port with saline solution, according to your hospital's policy. (Some hospitals require flushing the port with heparin solution first.)
• Clamp the extension set and remove the saline syringe.
• Connect the medication syringe to the extension set. Open the clamp and inject the drug, as ordered.
• Examine the skin surrounding the needle for signs of infiltration, such as swelling or tenderness. If you note these signs, stop the injection and intervene appropriately.
• When the injection is complete, clamp the extension set and remove the medication syringe.
• Open the clamp and flush with 5 ml of saline solution after each drug

injection to minimize drug incompatibility reactions.

• Flush with heparin solution, as your hospital's policy directs.

• Document the injection according to your hospital's policy, including the following information: the type and amount of medication injected; the time of the injection; the appearance of the site; the patient's tolerance of the procedure; and any pertinent nursing interventions.

Initiating a continuous infusion. After you've prepared the injection site and accessed the VAP, you can administer a continuous infusion, as ordered. Begin by gathering the following equipment: the prescribed I.V. solution or medication; an I.V. administration set; a filter, if ordered; an extension set; a clamp; a 10-ml syringe filled with saline solution; an antibacterial ointment (such as povidone-iodine ointment); adhesive tape; a sterile 2″ × 2″ gauze pad; sterile tape or adhesive skin closures; and a transparent semipermeable dressing. Now you're ready to administer the infusion following these steps:

• Remove all air from the extension set by priming it with an attached syringe of saline solution. Now attach the extension set to the noncoring needle.

• Flush the port system with saline solution. Clamp the extension set and remove the syringe.

• Connect the administration set, and secure the connections with tape, if necessary.

• Unclamp the extension set and begin the infusion.

• Apply a small amount of antibacterial ointment to the insertion site.

• Place the gauze pad under the needle hub if it doesn't lie flush with the skin. Secure the needle to the skin with sterile tape or adhesive

skin closures to help prevent needle dislodgment.

• Apply a transparent semipermeable dressing over the needle insertion site. (See *Continuous infusion: Securing the needle,* page 116.)

• Examine the site carefully for infiltration. If the patient complains of burning, stinging, or pain at the site, discontinue the infusion and intervene appropriately.

• When the solution container is empty, obtain a new I.V. solution container, as ordered, with primed I.V. tubing.

• Clamp the extension set and remove the old I.V. tubing.

• Attach the new I.V. tubing with the solution container to the extension set. Open the clamps, and adjust the infusion rate.

• Document the infusion according to your hospital's policy, including the following information: the type, amount, rate, and time of infusion; the patient's tolerance of the procedure; the appearance of the site; and any pertinent nursing interventions.

Maintaining infusion therapy

After the infusion therapy begins, your primary responsibility is to maintain it. This involves performing routine care measures, such as flushing the VAP with heparin solution. Maintaining therapy also involves being prepared to manage common equipment problems and patient complications. Finally, you'll need to discontinue therapy and establish a heparin lock to keep the device patent until it's needed again.

Continuous infusion: Securing the needle

When starting a continuous infusion, you must secure the right-angle non-coring needle to the skin as shown.

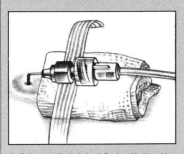

1. If the needle hub isn't flush with the skin, place a folded sterile dressing under the hub. Then apply adhesive skin closures across it.

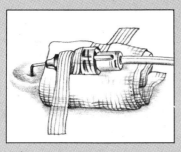

2. Secure the needle and tubing, using the chevron taping technique.

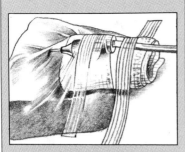

3. Apply a transparent semipermeable dressing over the entire site.

Routine care

If your patient is receiving a continuous or prolonged infusion, you'll need to flush the port with heparin solution after each use and change the dressing and needle every 5 to 7 days. You'll also need to change the tubing and solution, as you would for a long-term CV infusion.

If your patient's receiving an intermittent infusion, you'll need to flush the port periodically with heparin solution. During the course of therapy, you may have to obtain blood samples or clear a clotted VAP, as ordered.

Flushing a VAP with heparin solution. To help prevent clot formation you must flush the VAP with heparin solution after each use. When the VAP isn't being used, expect to flush it once every 4 weeks.

To flush the VAP, first gather the following equipment: a 22G non-coring needle with an extension set and a 10-ml syringe filled with 5 ml of sterile heparin flush solution (100 units/ml or recommended concentration). Prepare the injection site, as described above. Then follow these steps:
• Attach the 10-ml syringe with 5 ml of heparin flush solution to the non-coring needle and extension set. Apply gentle pressure to the plunger to remove all air from the set.
• Palpate the area over the port to locate it. Then access the port, as described above.
• Flush the VAP with the heparin solution.
• While stabilizing the VAP with two fingers, withdraw the non-coring needle.

Obtaining blood samples. You can obtain blood samples from an implanted VAP in two ways — with a syringe or with an evacuated tube

To obtain a blood sample with *a syringe*, first gather the following equipment: a 19G or 20G non-coring needle with an extension set, 10-ml syringe filled with 5 ml of saline solution, a 20-ml sterile syringe, a 20-ml sterile syringe filled with saline solution, blood sample tubes, and a sterile syringe filled with heparin flush solution.

Prepare the site, as described above. Then follow these steps:

• Attach the 10-ml syringe with 5 ml of saline solution to the non-coring needle and extension set. Remove all air from the set.

• Palpate the area over the port to locate it. Then access the port, as described above.

• Flush the VAP with 5 ml of saline solution.

• Withdraw at least 5 ml of blood; then clamp the extension set and discard the syringe.

• Connect a 20-ml sterile syringe to the extension set; unclamp the set.

• Aspirate the desired amount of blood into the 20-ml syringe.

• After obtaining the sample, clamp the extension set, remove the syringe, and attach a 20-ml syringe filled with saline solution. Unclamp the extension set.

• Immediately flush the VAP with 20 ml of saline solution. (*Note:* Solution concentrations and amounts may vary according to hospital policy.)

• Clamp the extension set, remove the saline syringe, and attach a sterile heparin-filled syringe. Perform the heparin flush procedure, as described above.

• Transfer the blood into appropriate blood sample tubes.

To obtain a blood sample using *an evacuated tube,* first gather the following equipment: a 19G or 20G non-coring needle with an extension set, a luer-lock injection cap, a 10-ml syringe of saline solution, alcohol or povidone-iodine swabs, an evacuated tube needle and holder (disposable tubes come with the needle already attached), blood sample tubes (label one "Discard"), a 20-ml sterile syringe filled with saline solution, and a sterile syringe filled with heparin flush solution. Prepare the site, as described above. Then follow these steps:

• Apply the evacuated tube needle to the tube's holder.

• Attach the luer-lock injection cap to the non-coring needle extension set, using sterile technique. Remove all air from the set with the saline-filled syringe.

• Palpate the area over the port to locate it. Then access the port, as described above.

• Flush the VAP with 5 ml of saline solution to ensure correct non-coring needle placement. Remove the saline syringe.

• Wipe the injection cap with an alcohol or povidone-iodine swab.

• Insert the evacuated tube needle into the injection cap.

• Insert the blood sample tube labeled "Discard" into the evacuated tube holder.

• Allow the tube to fill with blood (about 5 ml); remove the tube and discard.

• Insert another tube and allow it to fill with blood. Repeat this procedure until you obtain the necessary amount of blood.

• Remove the evacuated tube needle from the injection cap.

• Insert the 20-ml saline-filled syringe and immediately flush the VAP with 20 ml of saline solution; then remove the syringe.

• Next, attach the heparin-filled syringe and needle and perform the heparin flush procedure, as described above.

• After you've flushed the VAP with

saline solution and heparin, clamp the extension set.

• *Obtaining blood samples during therapy.* You may be ordered to obtain blood samples either before administering a bolus injection or during a continuous infusion. If you'll be administering a bolus injection, use the syringe method to obtain the blood sample, but don't flush with heparin solution.

If the patient is already receiving a continuous infusion, shut off the infusion and clamp the extension set. Then disconnect the extension set, maintaining aseptic technique. Follow the procedure for obtaining a blood sample with a syringe, up to and including the saline flush procedure. After the catheter is flushed with saline solution, clamp the extension set and remove the syringe. Reconnect the I.V. extension set. Then, unclamp it and adjust the flow rate.

Administering a fibrinolytic. If clotting threatens to occlude the VAP, the doctor may order a fibrinolytic agent, such as urokinase, to clear the catheter. Because such agents increase the risk of bleeding, urokinase may be contraindicated in patients who've had surgery within the past 10 days; who have active internal bleeding, such as GI bleeding; or who've experienced central nervous system damage, such as infarction, hemorrhage, trauma, surgery, or primary or metastatic disease within the past 2 months.

To clear the VAP, gather the following equipment: a 22G non-coring needle with an extension set; a 1-ml syringe filled with urokinase (5,000 I.U. in 1-ml sterile water is the usual dosage for clotted catheters); an empty 10-ml syringe; a 5-ml syringe and a 10-ml syringe, both filled with saline solution; and a sterile syringe filled with heparin flush solution. Prepare the site as described, then follow these steps:

• Palpate the area over the port and access the VAP as described above. Check for blood return.

• Flush the VAP with 5 ml of saline solution and clamp the extension tubing.

• Attach the 1-ml syringe and unclamp the extension tubing. Then instill the urokinase solution, using a gentle pull-push motion on the syringe plunger to mix the solution within the VAP and the catheter.

• Clamp the extension set.

• Leave the solution in place for 15 minutes.

• Attach an empty 10-ml syringe.

• Unclamp the extension set and aspirate the urokinase and clot with the 10-ml syringe.

• If the clot can't be aspirated, wait 5 minutes and try again. You can safely instill urokinase solution as many as three times in a 4-hour period, if the patient's platelet count is greater than 20,000/mm^3. Repeat the procedure only once in a 4-hour period, if the patient's platelet count is less than 20,000/mm^3.

• After the blockage has been cleared, flush the catheter with at least 10 ml of saline solution.

• Flush the catheter with heparin solution, as described above.

Documenting the infusion. Record your assessment findings and interventions according to your hospital policy. Include the following information: the type, amount, rate, and duration of the infusion; the appearance of the site; the development of problems, if any, and the steps taken to resolve them; needle and dressing changes for continuous infusions; blood samples obtained, including the type and amount; and patient teaching topics covered.

Managing common VAP problems

To maintain a vascular access port (VAP), you must be able to handle common problems. This chart outlines problems you may encounter, their possible causes, and the appropriate nursing interventions.

POSSIBLE CAUSE	NURSING INTERVENTIONS
Inability to flush VAP or withdraw blood	
• Kinked tubing or closed clamp	• Check tubing or clamp.
• Catheter lodged against vessel wall	• Reposition patient. • Teach patient to change his position to free catheter from the vessel wall. • Raise the arm that's on the same side as catheter. • Roll patient to the opposite side. • Have patient cough, sit up, or take a deep breath. • Infuse 10 ml of saline solution into catheter. • Regain access to catheter or VAP, using a new sterile needle.
• Incorrect needle placement • Needle not advanced through septum	• Regain access to device. • Teach home care patient to push down firmly on non-coring needle device in septum and to verify needle position by aspirating for a blood return.
• Clot formation	• Assess patency by trying to flush VAP while the patient changes position. • Notify doctor; obtain order for urokinase instillation. • Teach patient to recognize clot formation, to notify the doctor if it occurs, and to avoid forcibly flushing VAP.
• Kinked catheter, catheter migration, port rotation	• Notify doctor immediately. • Tell patient to notify doctor if he has difficulty using VAP.
Inability to palpate VAP	
• Deeply implanted port	• Note portal chamber scar. • Use deep palpation technique. • Ask another nurse to try locating VAP. • Use a 1½" or 2" (3.8 to 5.1 cm) non-coring needle to gain access to VAP.

Correcting common problems

Besides performing routine care measures, you must be prepared to handle several common problems that may arise during an infusion with a VAP. These common problems include an inability to flush the VAP, an inability to withdraw blood from it, and an inability to palpate it. (See *Managing common VAP problems.*)

Patients with special needs

Generally, the procedures for implanting and maintaining a VAP are the same for pediatric and elderly patients as for adult patients. With pediatric patients, however, general anesthesia is typically used during implantation.

A home care patient, however, needs thorough teaching about procedures and follow-up visits from a home care nurse to ensure his safety and the success of his treatment. If the patient will be accessing the port himself, explain that the most uncomfortable part of the procedure is the actual insertion of the needle into the skin. Once the needle has penetrated the skin, the patient will feel mostly pressure. Eventually, the skin over the port will become desensitized from frequent needle punctures. Until then, the patient may want to use a topical anesthetic.

Stress the importance of pushing the needle into the port until he feels the needle bevel touch the back of the port. Many patients tend to stop short of the back of the port, leaving the needle bevel in the rubber septum.

Complications of therapy

A patient who has a VAP faces risks similar to those associated with CV catheters. These include complications such as infection and infiltration. (See *Risks of VAP therapy*.)

Discontinuing therapy

To discontinue therapy, you'll need to stop the infusion and establish a heparin lock, which maintains the patency of the VAP. Then you'll need to remove the non-coring needle from the port.

Creating a heparin lock. To keep the VAP from becoming occluded, you must fill it with heparin flush solution after each use. To create a heparin lock, first gather the following equipment: a 10-ml syringe with saline solution, a 20G needle, 10-ml syringe filled with 5 ml of sterile heparin flush solution (100 units/ml), a luer-lock injection cap, and alcohol or povidone-iodine swabs. Then follow these steps:
• Shut off the infusion.
• Clamp the extension set and remove the I.V. tubing.
• Attach the luer-lock injection cap to the extension set.
• Wipe the cap with an alcohol or povidone-iodine swab.
• Attach the needle to the syringe filled with saline solution.
• Unclamp the extension set and flush the device with the saline solution. Remove the saline syringe.
• Attach the needle to the heparin syringe and wipe the cap with an alcohol or povidone-iodine swab.
• Flush the VAP with heparin solution and clamp the extension set until its next use.

Removing the non-coring needle. After you've flushed the port with heparin solution, you can remove the non-coring needle. To do so, follow these steps:
• Put a sterile glove on your non-dominant hand.
• Place the index and middle finger of your gloved hand on either side of the port septum, almost touching the needle.
• Stabilize the port by pressing down with the two fingers on either side of the port septum. Maintain this pressure until the needle is removed.
• Using your ungloved (dominant) hand, grasp the non-coring needle at its bend and pull it straight out of the port.
• Clean the site with an alcohol swab, and apply a dressing as indicated.

COMPLICATIONS

Risks of VAP therapy

The following chart lists some common complications of vascular access port (VAP) therapy, as well as their signs and symptoms, causes, and the appropriate nursing interventions and prevention measures.

SIGNS AND SYMPTOMS	POSSIBLE CAUSES	NURSING INTERVENTIONS
Site infection or skin breakdown		
• Erythema and warmth at the port site • Oozing or purulent drainage at port site or VAP pocket • Fever	• Infected incision or VAP pocket • Poor postoperative healing	• Assess site daily for redness; note any drainage. • Notify doctor. • Administer antibiotics, as ordered. • Apply warm soaks for 20 minutes four times a day. *Prevention:* • Teach patient to inspect for and report any redness, swelling, drainage, or skin breakdown at the port site.
Extravasation		
• Burning sensation or swelling in subcutaneous tissue	• Needle dislodged into subcutaneous tissue • Needle incorrectly placed in VAP • Needle position not confirmed; needle pulled out of septum	• Don't remove needle. • Stop infusion. • Notify doctor; prepare to administer antidote, if ordered. *Prevention:* • Teach patient how to gain access to the device; verify placement of the device; and secure the needle before initiating the infusion.
Thrombosis		
• Inability to flush port or administer infusion	• Frequent blood sampling • Infusion of packed red blood cells (PRBCs)	• Notify doctor; obtain order to administer urokinase. *Prevention:* • Flush VAP thoroughly right after obtaining blood sample. • Administer PRBCs as a piggyback with saline solution and use an infusion pump; flush with saline solution between units.
Fibrin sheath formation		
• Blocked port and catheter lumen • Inability to flush port or administer infusion	• Adherence of platelets to catheter	*Prevention:* • Use port only to infuse fluids and medications; don't use to obtain blood samples. • Administer only compatible substances through port.

If no more infusions are scheduled, be sure to remind the patient of the need for a heparin flush in 4 weeks. Finally, document the removal of the infusion needle, the status of the site, the use of the heparin flush, your patient-teaching efforts, and any problems you encountered and resolved.

Suggested readings

Bartlett, K., et al. "Venous Access Devices: Appropriate for Home Use," *Home Healthcare Nurse* 8(2):38-41, March-April 1990.

Brown, J.M. "Evaluation of Surecath Access Devices," *Journal of Intravenous Nursing* 12(5):298-301, September/October 1989.

Hadaway, L.C., "Evaluation and Use of Advance I.V. Technology: Central Venous Access Devices," Part I. *Journal of Intravenous Nursing* 12(2):73-82, March-April 1989.

Hagle, M. "Implantable Devices for Chemotherapy: Access and Delivery," *Seminar in Oncology Nursing* 3(2):96-105, May 1987.

Handy, C.M. "Vascular Access Devices, Hospital to Home Care," *Journal of Intravenous Nursing* 12 (Suppl.):S10-S17, January/February 1989.

Hower, D.K. "Blood Samples Made Simple: Using Special I.V. Lines at Home," *Nursing87* 17(7):56-58, July 1987.

Newman, L.N. "A Side by Side Look at Two Venous Access Devices," *American Journal of Nursing* 89(6):826-35, June 1989.

Viall, C.D. "Your Complete Guide to Central Venous Catheters," *Nursing90* 20(2):34-41, February 1990.

Weinstein, S.M. "Thrombolytic Therapy," *NITA* 9(1):31-35, January/February 1986.

5

I.V. MEDICATIONS

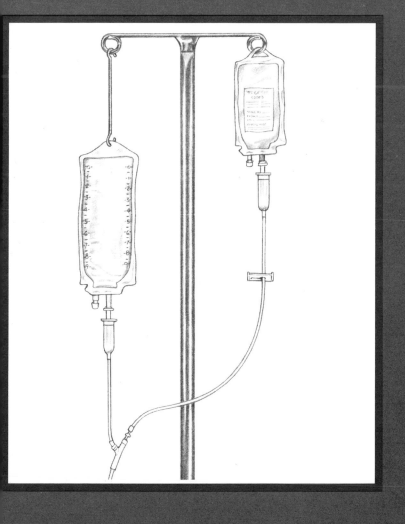

Hospitalized patients receive about 40% of their medications by the I.V. route. This includes medications given by direct injection, intermittent infusion, continuous infusion, and specialized devices such as the patient-controlled analgesia (PCA) device.

To give I.V. drugs by these various methods, you need to understand the principles and procedures explained in this chapter. The first section covers the basics of I.V. medication therapy, including indications, advantages, and disadvantages. The next section explains preparation for I.V. drug administration. You'll review how to calculate dosages and administration rates, prepare medications, and select the proper equipment. The third section tells you how to initiate therapy, using direct injection, intermittent infusion, and continuous infusion. You'll also review how PCA devices work. The final section deals with maintaining therapy — specifically how to monitor patients for common complications, how to care for pediatric and elderly patients, and what to teach patients who will continue their therapy at home.

Basics of I.V. medication therapy

A doctor may order an I.V. medication when:
• a patient needs a rapid therapeutic effect
• the medication can't be absorbed by the GI tract — either because it has a high molecular weight or it's unstable in gastric juices
• the patient should receive nothing by mouth and an irritating drug would cause pain or tissue damage if given I.M. or S.C.
• a controlled administration rate is needed.

Advantages
Compared with the oral, S.C., and I.M. routes, the I.V. route has many advantages. It provides immediate drug action by producing therapeutic blood levels rapidly. Thus, it's the preferred route in emergencies. The I.V. route also eliminates absorption problems, allows for accurate titration, and causes the patient less discomfort.

No absorption problems. With S.C. and I.M. drugs, absorption may be erratic. And some oral drugs prove unstable in gastric juices and digestive enzymes. Also, many oral drugs are absorbed slowly — and absorption may be erratic or incomplete. In part, that's because oral drugs must pass through the liver, where significant amounts are metabolized and eliminated before they reach the bloodstream. This metabolism, known as first-pass metabolism, may be so rapid and extensive (in the case of lidocaine, for example) that it precludes oral administration.

I.V. drugs, on the other hand, go directly into the patient's circulation, rapidly achieving therapeutic blood levels. This difference in absorption explains why for some drugs, such as propranolol, I.V. doses are much smaller than oral doses.

Accurate titration. Because absorption isn't a factor with I.V. administration, you can accurately titrate medication doses by adjusting the concentration and the administration rate.

Less discomfort. Rapid delivery of some I.V. drugs can cause venous irritation. But the veins have a much higher pain threshold than muscle or subcutaneous tissue. So I.V. administration avoids the pain and discomfort associated with I.M. and S.C. injections. Besides, you can sometimes reduce venous irritation by further diluting an I.V. solution. You can't substantially dilute S.C. or I.M. drugs because the volume must remain small.

Other advantages. The I.V. route provides an alternative when you can't use the oral route — for example, when your patient is unconscious or uncooperative or can take nothing by mouth. If an adverse reaction occurs, the I.V. route allows you to stop drug delivery immediately. With other routes, absorption would continue until the drug was physically removed — by vomiting, for instance.

Disadvantages

Like all administration routes, the I.V. route has certain disadvantages. These include solution and drug incompatibilities, poor vascular access in some patients, and immediate adverse reactions.

Incompatibility. Before mixing an I.V. drug solution, make sure the drugs, diluent, and solution are compatible. If you're not sure, check with the hospital pharmacist. Remember, an incompatibility may occur when you mix drugs in a syringe or solution container or when you deliver an I.V. drug piggyback through an existing I.V. line.

The commonly used I.V. solutions are compatible with most I.V. drugs. But the more complex the solution, the greater the risk of incompatibility. An I.V. solution containing divalent cations (such as Ca^{++}) has a higher incidence of incompatibility. So lactated Ringer's solution and Ringer's injection solution, for example, can present mixing problems. These problems are also common with alcohol, mannitol, and nutritional solutions.

When a drug loses more than 10% of its potency, it's considered incompatible with whatever caused the loss of potency. Drug incompatibility may result from:
• binding of two drugs. For example, when mixed in the same container, gentamicin sulfate and carbenicillin disodium form a complex, resulting in a substantial loss of gentamicin's activity.
• a physical alteration such as precipitation, color change, or gas formation. For instance, mixing heparin sodium with gentamicin sulfate causes immediate precipitation.
• a chemical change in the drug solution. When erythromycin lactobionate is added to dextrose 5% in water (D_5W), the low pH of the solution causes decomposition of the antibiotic.

Other factors can affect incompatibility, including the order in which drugs are mixed, drug concentrations, contact time, temperature, light, and pH. (See *Factors affecting drug incompatibility,* page 126.)

Poor vascular access. In an emergency, you may find that normally accessible veins have collapsed from vasoconstriction or hypovolemia. Venipuncture may also be difficult in patients who require frequent or prolonged I.V. therapy. You may find that they've developed small, scarred, inaccessible veins from repeated venipunctures or infusions of irritating drugs.

If peripheral venous access isn't possible, the doctor may use a

Factors affecting drug incompatibility

The term *incompatibility* refers to an undesirable chemical or physical reaction between a drug and a solution or between two or more drugs. These factors can affect the compatibility of an I.V. drug solution.

Order of mixing
This will be a concern when you're adding more than one drug to an I.V. solution. Chemical changes occur after you add each drug. So a drug that's compatible with the I.V. solution alone may be incompatible with the mixture of I.V. solution and another drug. Changing the order in which you mix the drugs may avoid incompatibility.

Drug concentration
The higher the drug concentration, the more likely an incompatibility will develop. The purpose of gently inverting the container after adding each drug is to evenly disperse it throughout the solution, preventing a high concentration buildup. You should do this before starting an infusion and before adding another drug to the container.

Contact time
The longer two or more drugs are together, the more likely an incompatibility will occur. You should know if two drugs are immediately incompatible before deciding how to give them.

Suppose, for example, your patient is receiving a continuous heparin infusion, and gentamicin sulfate is ordered. Because these two drugs have an immediate incompatibility, you shouldn't piggyback the gentamicin into the heparin solution. If you do, your patient won't receive a therapeutic dose of gentamicin.

Temperature
Higher temperatures promote chemical reactions. So the higher the temperature of an admixture, the greater the risk of incompatibility. For this reason, you should prepare the admixture right before administering it, or refrigerate it until needed.

Light
Prolonged exposure to light can affect the stability of certain drugs. Nitrofurantoin and amphotericin B, for example, must be protected from light during administration to maintain their stability.

pH
Generally, drugs and solutions that will be mixed should have similar pH values to avoid incompatibility. You'll find the pH of each I.V. solution listed on the manufacturer's label. You'll find the pH of each drug on the package insert.

central vein, frequently the subclavian. He probably won't use the femoral vein because inadvertent venipuncture of the femoral artery and subsequent intra-arterial injection can cause arterial spasm and gangrene.

If venipuncture isn't possible, drugs are usually given I.M. or S.C. However, these routes can be used only if the volume is small and the drugs cause little or no tissue irritation.

Adverse reactions. Because I.V. drugs quickly produce high blood levels, severe adverse reactions may occur immediately. The particular adverse reactions will depend on the drug.

Hypersensitivity to I.V. drugs, although uncommon, can occur either immediately or at any time after administration. Keep in mind that if a patient is hypersensitive to a particular drug, he may be hypersensitive to other chemically similar drugs. This is known as cross-sensitivity. The most severe hypersensitivity reaction is anaphylaxis. The drugs most likely to produce this reaction include penicillin and its synthetic derivatives.

Your patient may also suffer an adverse reaction from the preservative in the drug or I.V. solution. Large amounts of benzyl alcohol, for example, may cause seizures in neonates. And sulfites, another type of preservative, can cause sensitivity reactions in some people — particularly those with asthma.

You may also encounter patients who have an inherent inability to tolerate certain chemicals. They can experience another kind of adverse reaction, called an idiosyncratic reaction. For example, in a particular patient, a tranquilizer may cause excitation rather than sedation.

Preparing to administer I.V. medications

Before you can give an I.V. medication to your patient, you may have to calculate the drug dosage and the administration rate. You'll also need to prepare the medication for delivery and select the equipment.

Calculating I.V. drug dosages
Often, you'll be responsible for preparing the ordered dosage and for verifying that the dosage is within the recommended range.

With some drugs (immune globulin I.V., for instance), the dosage will be based on the patient's weight in kilograms. So you'll have to first convert his weight from pounds to kilograms. To do this, simply divide the number of pounds by 2.2. Remember, 2.2 lb = 1 kg.

With other drugs (such as chemotherapeutic agents), the dosage will be based on the patient's body surface area. You can use one of two simple methods to determine this area. (See *Using a body surface area slide rule,* page 128, and *Using a nomogram,* page 129.)

Calculating administration rates
Typically, you'll receive an order for I.V. medication that tells you how many milliliters to give over a period of time — for instance, 1,000 ml of 5% dextrose in 0.45% sodium chloride every 8 hours. To make sure you deliver the drug solution evenly, you need to determine how many milliliters to give in 1 hour. So just divide the total volume by the number of hours. In this case, you'd divide 1,000 by 8 to find that you must give 125 ml/hour.

Additional orders. Often, additional I.V. orders will affect your calculations. Suppose the patient who's receiving the 1,000 ml of 5% dextrose in 0.45% sodium chloride every 8 hours is also receiving gentamicin 80 mg every 8 hours by intermittent infusion. You won't deliver the primary solution while administering the gentamicin, but you still need to give the 1,000 ml in 8 hours, as ordered. To find the hourly flow rate for the primary solution, first subtract the time needed to give the gentamicin from the total time period. If you're giving the gentamicin over 1 hour, you'd have 7 hours left to give

Using a body surface area slide rule

To calculate your patient's body surface area with a special slide rule, such as the one below, place the patient's weight directly opposite his height. Then read the body surface area in square meters (m²) at the arrow.

On the slide rule below, you can see that a patient weighing 110 lb with a height of 5′3″ has a body surface area of 1.5 m²

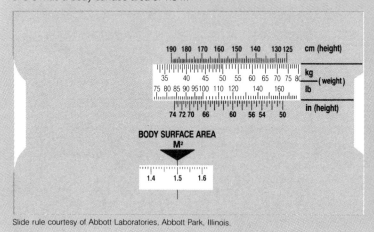

Slide rule courtesy of Abbott Laboratories, Abbott Park, Illinois.

the primary solution. Now, divide 1,000 by 7 to find that you must deliver the primary solution at a rate of 143 ml/hour.

Equipment considerations. Your calculations may also depend on the delivery equipment. If you're using an infusion pump, simply dial the desired ml/hour rate. But if you're using a controller or an administration set, you have to convert ml/hour to drops/minute (gtt/minute).

To do this, you must know the number of drops per milliliter that the particular I.V. tubing delivers. All manufacturers make microdrip tubings with a 60 gtt/ml factor, but macrodrip tubings vary. To find gtt/ml information, check the product wrapper or box, then use this formula: gtt/ml of I.V. tubing ÷ 60 × ml/hour needed = gtt/minute.

Preparing medications

Most I.V. drug solutions will be prepared in the pharmacy by pharmacists or pharmacy technicians. But in some situations, you'll have to prepare I.V. drug solutions yourself before administering them.

Ensuring safety. When you're preparing a medication for I.V. administration, be sure to check the expiration date on the drug and the diluent and look for any special diluent requirements. Note whether the drug requires filtration. Also, inspect the drug, diluent, and solution for particles and cloudiness. After reconstitution, again be sure to check for any visible signs of incompatibility in the admixture. Remember, incompatibility is more likely with drugs or I.V. solutions that have a high or low pH. Most

Using a nomogram

To estimate body surface area with a nomogram, find your patient's weight in the right column and his height in the left column. Mark these two points, then draw a line between them. The point where the line intersects the middle column gives you the surface area in square meters (m²).

On this nomogram, the patient's height is 5'3" and weight is 110 lb. A straight line drawn between the two columns intersects the center column at 1.50. That tells you this patient's body surface area is 1.5 m².

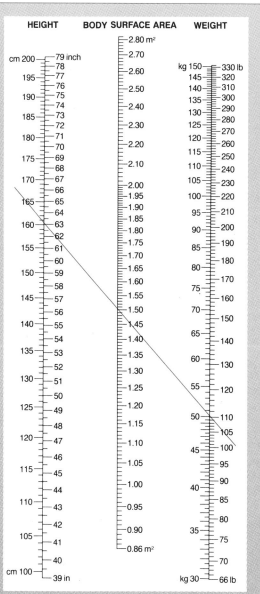

drugs are moderately acidic, but some are alkaline, including heparin, aminophylline, ampicillin sodium, and sodium bicarbonate.

If you're mixing a drug in a minibag or minibottle of 0.9% sodium chloride (normal saline solution) or D_5W, you may be able to use the solution in the minicontainer as the diluent. But be sure to inspect it, and discard any solution that appears cloudy or contains particles. Some solutions change color after several hours. If you're not sure whether to use a discolored solution, ask the pharmacist.

Maintain aseptic technique. Always wash your hands before mixing, and avoid contaminating any part of the vial, ampule, syringe, needle, or container that must remain sterile. When you're inserting the needle into and withdrawing it from the vial, make sure the needle tip doesn't touch an unsterile part of the vial or inadvertently puncture your finger. To keep your hands steady, brace one against the other while you're inserting and withdrawing the needle.

When drawing up the drug before adding it to the primary solution, make sure you use a syringe large enough to hold the entire dose. The needle should be at least 1″ long to penetrate the inner seal of the port on an I.V. bag. In many hospitals, practitioners use a 5-micron needle for mixing drug powder or withdrawing drugs from glass ampules.

Reconstituting drugs. Many I.V. drugs are supplied in powder form and require reconstitution with such diluents as normal saline solution, sterile water for injection, or D_5W. Note any specific manufacturer's instructions about the appropriate type or amount of diluent. Some

drugs should be reconstituted with diluents that don't have preservatives.

To reconstitute a drug powder, follow these steps:
- Draw up the amount and type of diluent specified by the manufacturer.
- Clean the rubber stopper of the drug vial with an alcohol swab, using aseptic technique.
- Insert the needle connected to the syringe of diluent into the stopper at a 45- to 60-degree angle. This minimizes coring or breaking off rubber pieces, which would then float inside the vial.
- Inject the diluent.
- Mix thoroughly by gently inverting the vial. If the drug doesn't dissolve within a few seconds, let it stand for 10 to 30 minutes. If necessary, invert the vial several times to dissolve the drug. Don't shake vigorously (unless directed) because some drugs may froth.

Diluting liquid drugs. Liquid drugs come in single-dose ampules, multidose vials, prefilled syringes, and disposable cartridges with attached needles. Liquid drugs don't need reconstitution, but they often require dilution. When diluting such a drug, remember that all liquid drug containers are overfilled. So be sure to withdraw *only* the prescribed amount.

Using specialized containers. Some drugs come in *double-chambered vials* that contain powder in the lower chamber and a diluent in the upper one. To combine these contents, apply pressure to the rubber stopper on top of the vial to dislodge the rubber plug separating the compartments. The diluent will then mix with the drug in the bottom chamber.

Additive vials of drug can be attached directly to administration tubing. If the vial contains a drug powder, first reconstitute it. Then you can infuse the drug solution directly from the vial.

Adding a drug. To add a drug to an *I.V. bottle*, first clean the rubber stopper or latex diaphragm with alcohol. Then insert the needle (either 19G or 20G) of the medication-filled syringe into the center of the stopper or diaphragm and inject the drug. Next, invert the bottle at least twice so you ensure thorough mixing. Now remove the latex diaphragm and insert the administration spike.

To add a drug to a *plastic I.V. bag,* insert the needle of the medication-filled syringe into the clean latex medication port and inject the drug. (The needle should be 19G or 20G and 1″ long; a short needle won't pierce the inner port seal, and a small-volume additive such as insulin will remain in the port.) After injecting the drug, grasp the top and bottom of the bag and quickly invert it twice. Don't squeeze or shake the bag.

• *Adding to an infusing solution.* If you have a choice, don't add a drug to an I.V. solution that's already infusing because of the risk of altering the drug concentration. But if you must add a drug, be sure the primary solution container contains enough solution to provide adequate dilution. To add the drug, clamp the I.V. tubing and take down the container. Then with the container upright, add the drug.

If you're adding the drug to a bottle, clean the rubber stopper with an alcohol swab, insert the needle through the stopper, and inject the drug. If you're adding the drug to an I.V. bag, clean the rubber injection port with an alcohol swab before you inject the drug.

After injecting the drug into the container, invert it several times to ensure thorough mixing and prevent a bolus effect.

Labeling solution containers. Containers prepared in the pharmacy will have a label showing the patient's full name and room number, the date, the name and amount of the I.V. solution and drugs, and other vital information. If you prepare the drug solution, be sure to label the container with this information. Also, note the date and time you mixed the drug solution and sign or initial the label. Make sure your label doesn't cover the manufacturer's label.

If you use a time-strip, label it with the patient's name and room number and the infusion rate (in ml/hour, gtt/minute, or both).

Selecting the equipment

The type of equipment you choose will depend on how you'll be administering the drug. The primary choice you'll make will concern the type of tubing.

Here are several questions to consider:

1. Do you need a pump or controller to deliver the particular drug? Hospitals usually have policies regarding the use of these devices. Pumps and controllers, most of which still require specific administration sets, are frequently used when you need a precise or very low infusion rate. They're also used when you're administering fluids or admixtures through a central venous catheter.

2. What's the ordered drip rate and what's your hospital's policy on using macrodrip and microdrip tubings? Many policies require mi-

2 Italian Sais

EQUIPMENT

A needle-free system

You can now piggyback drugs or additional I.V. solutions into a primary line without using a needle. Instead, you'll use a system that consists of a blunt-tipped plastic insertion device and a rubber injection port. The port may be part of a special administration set or an adapter for existing administration sets. This rubber injection port has a pre-established slit that can open and reseal immediately.

This system can greatly reduce the risk of accidental needle-stick injuries. Of course, the system can't eliminate all such injuries because it can't be used to perform venipunctures.

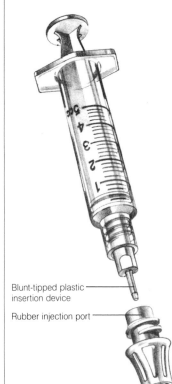

Blunt-tipped plastic insertion device

Rubber injection port

crodrip tubing when the infusion rate is less than 63 ml/hour.

3. Is your patient going to receive intermittent drug infusions as well as the primary drug solution? If so, you may need a primary tubing that has an injection port close to the drip chamber and a backcheck valve that'll automatically shut off the primary solution when the secondary solution is infusing.

4. Is your patient going to receive a simultaneous infusion of a secondary drug solution? If so, you'll need tubing that has an injection port close to the venipuncture device because you don't want to stop the primary infusion.

5. Does the drug solution require special tubing? Tubing without polyvinylchloride is recommended for certain drugs, such as nitroglycerin.

6. Will you be using a needle-free system? If so, be sure to use the appropriate administration set or a special adapter. (See *A needle-free system.*)

7. Is the solution container made of glass or plastic? If you're using a glass container, you'll need vented I.V. tubing. Use nonvented tubing for a collapsible plastic bag.

8. Is your patient an infant or a small child? Many hospitals have policies that permit only volume-control sets for such patients. These devices limit the volume available to the patient and decrease the risk of inadvertent fluid overload.

Initiating therapy

You can administer I.V. medications by direct injection, intermittent infusion, or continuous infusion. Each of these methods has certain indications, advantages, and disadvantages. (See *Comparing administration methods*, pages 134 and 135.) You may also administer an I.V. medication using a specialized device, such as the PCA device.

Before you administer I.V. medication by any of the methods mentioned, confirm the patient's identity by checking his name, room number, and bed number on his wristband (see *Remember the five rights*). Also, check his history for allergies and explain the procedure to him.

Be sure you know some key information about the drug you'll be giving. For instance, you should know the normal dosage, expected effects, adverse reactions, contraindications, and drug interactions. If you're unfamiliar with the drug and don't have access to the drug package insert or a drug reference book, ask your pharmacist any drug-related questions.

Follow the Centers for Disease Control (CDC) guidelines to protect yourself and your patient from infection. This means wearing gloves (and possibly gowns and masks) when exposed to body fluids.

After you administer the drug, always document your actions, noting the date and time, drug and dosage, access site, duration of administration, patient's response, and your name or initials.

Direct injection
Commonly called I.V. push, direct injection can be administered as a single dose (bolus) or intermittent multiple doses directly into a vein or through an existing infusion line.

Direct injection often produces adverse reactions because of the high drug concentrations. This method also exerts more pressure on the vein than other methods,

CHECKLIST

Remember the five rights

Before you administer an I.V. drug to a patient, make sure you check the five rights:
☐ right drug
☐ right patient
☐ right time
☐ right dosage
☐ right route.
    At the same time, make sure the patient understands the medication he'll be receiving. Also, make sure he knows he has the right to refuse to take the medication.

posing a greater risk of infiltration in patients with fragile veins.

Most drugs must be given over a specific time period when using direct injection. To avoid speed shock, don't administer any drug in less than 1 minute — unless the order states otherwise or the patient is in cardiac or respiratory arrest.

Remember, too, that systemic edema, pulmonary congestion, decreased cardiac output, and reduced urine output, renal flow, and glomerular filtration can all cause decreased drug tolerance. If your patient has any of these conditions, longer injection times or greater drug dilution may be required.

Injection into a vein. To inject a drug directly into a vein, you need a winged small-vein needle, a syringe with medication, a 3-ml syringe filled with saline solution, an alcohol swab, a tourniquet, gloves, tape, and a sterile pressure dressing. You should use the winged needle for I.V. push because it can be inserted quickly and easily. This makes it ideal for a patient on a weekly

(Text continues on page 136.)

Comparing administration methods

You can administer I.V. medications in several ways. This chart gives you the indications, advantages, and disadvantages of the common methods.

METHOD & INDICATIONS	ADVANTAGES	DISADVANTAGES
Direct injection		
Into a vein (no infusion line) • When a nonvesicant drug with low risk of immediate adverse reaction is required for a patient with no other I.V. needs (for example, outpatients requiring I.V. contrast injections for radiologic examinations or cancer patients receiving chemotherapeutic agents).	• Eliminates risk of complications from indwelling venipuncture device. • Eliminates inconvenience of indwelling venipuncture device.	• Can only be given by doctor or specially certified nurse. • Requires venipuncture, which can cause patient anxiety. • Requires two syringes – one to administer medication and one to flush the vein after administration. • Risk of infiltration from steel needle. • Can't dilute drug or interrupt delivery when irritation occurs. • Risk of clotting with the administration of a drug over a long period and with a small volume.
Through existing infusion line • When drug required is incompatible with I.V. solution and must be given as bolus injection for therapeutic effect. • When patient requires immediate high blood levels (for example, regular insulin, 50% dextrose, atropine, and antihistamines). • In emergencies, when the drug must be given quickly for immediate effect.	• Doesn't require time or authorization to perform venipuncture because the vein is already accessed. • Doesn't require needle puncture, which can cause patient anxiety. • Allows use of I.V. solution to test patency of venipuncture device before drug administration. • Allows continued venous access in case of adverse reactions. • Reduces risk of infiltration with vesicant drugs because most continuous infusions are started with an over-the-needle catheter.	• Carries the same inconveniences and risks of complications associated with indwelling venipuncture device.

Comparing administration methods *(continued)*

METHOD & INDICATIONS	ADVANTAGES	DISADVANTAGES
Intermittent infusion		
Piggyback method • Often used with drugs given over short periods at varying intervals (for example, antibiotics and gastric-secretion inhibitors).	• Avoids multiple needle injections required by I.M. route. • Permits repeated administration of drugs through single I.V. site. • Provides high drug blood levels for short periods without causing drug toxicity.	• May cause periods when drug blood level becomes too low to be clinically effective (for example when peak-and-trough times aren't considered in the medication order).
Heparin lock • When patient requires constant venous access, but not a continuous infusion.	• Provides venous access for patients with fluid restrictions. • Provides better patient mobility between doses. • Preserves veins by reducing venipunctures. • Lower cost.	• Requires close monitoring during administration so device can be flushed on completion. • Heparin flush can't be used if patient has heparin sensitivity. • Cost can rise rapidly when using device for several drugs because of equipment required.
Volume-control set • When patient requires low volume of fluid.	• Requires only one large-volume container. Prevents fluid overload from a runaway infusion. • Chamber can be reused.	• High cost. • High risk of contamination. • If set doesn't contain membrane to block air passage when empty, you must close flow clamp when the set empties.
Continuous infusion		
Through primary line • When continuous serum levels are needed and there's little chance infusion will be stopped abruptly.	• Maintains steady serum levels. • Less risk of rapid shock and vein irritation from large volume of fluid diluting the drug.	• Risk of incompatibility increases with drug contact time. • Patient connected to an I.V. system, restricting his mobility. • Increased risk of undetected infiltration because slow infusion makes it difficult to see an increased infiltration area.
Through secondary line • When patient requires continuous infusion of two or more compatible admixtures administered at different rates. • When there's moderate-to-high chance you'll have to abruptly stop one admixture without infusing the drug remaining in the I.V. tubing.	• Primary infusion and each secondary infusion can be given at different rates. • Primary line may be totally shut off and kept on standby to maintain venous access in case secondary line must be abruptly stopped. • Short contact time before infusion may allow the administration of incompatible admixtures – something not possible with long contact time.	• Eliminates use of drugs with immediate incompatibility. • Increased risk of vein irritation or phlebitis from increased number of drugs. • Use of multiple I.V. systems (for example primary lines with secondary lines attached), especially with electronic pumps or controllers, can create physical barriers to patient care and limit patient mobility.

EQUIPMENT

Intermittent infusions: Special devices

You may be asked to administer medications using any of the following devices.

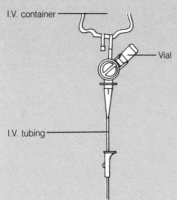

I.V. container

Vial

I.V. tubing

Special tubing

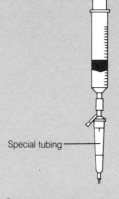

Controlled release infusion system (CRIS). Place this device between the I.V. container and the tubing, then attach the drug vial to its side, as shown. The I.V. fluid passes into the device where it mixes with the drug from the vial to deliver a controlled amount of medication to the patient.

Secondary syringe converter (ACCUSAVE). This special administration set converts any syringe into a piggyback container. The tubing connects to the syringe instead of a bag or bottle. You use the same procedure you would with a minibag, substituting the syringe for the minibag.

or monthly nonvesicant chemotherapy regimen.

To inject a drug directly into a vein, apply the tourniquet and clean the I.V. site with an alcohol swab. Then follow these steps:
• Connect the syringe with medication to the small-vein needle and push the plunger to remove the air.
• Select the largest suitable vein to allow for rapid dilution. Put on gloves and insert the needle in the vein with the bevel up.
• Withdraw a small amount of blood to confirm needle placement.
• Release the tourniquet.
• Place a short narrow strip of tape over each needle wing to secure

the needle during administration.
• Inject the drug at an even rate, as ordered.
• Gently withdraw the plunger at frequent intervals to reconfirm needle placement and ensure the delivery of all medication.
• Observe your patient for any signs of adverse reactions during and after the injection.
• Disconnect the medication syringe from the small-vein needle. Attach the syringe filled with saline to the needle and flush the line to ensure the delivery of all medication.
• Remove the venipuncture device and immediately place a sterile pressure dressing over the I.V. site.

Syringe pumps. Battery-operated mini-infusion syringe pumps can be used to infuse small volumes intermittently or continuously. You'll find them especially useful for pediatric patients.

The syringe and microbore tubing replace the minibag and piggyback tubing to deliver a precise volume over the prescribed time.

The major disadvantage of the syringe pump is that you need tubing to connect it to the venipuncture device. So when you give a small-volume dose, a portion of the drug remains in the tubing. You can help limit the amount of drug remaining by using small-volume tubing. (Standard I.V. tubing holds 1.9 ml/foot; small-volume tubing has a smaller lumen and holds only 0.06 ml/foot.)

Also remember syringe pumps don't have air detectors. So be sure to eliminate all air from the syringe, tubing, and needle. Use luer-locks and tape for all connections. This helps prevent partial disconnections that could cause an air infusion or drug leak.

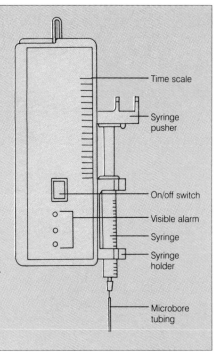

Time scale

Syringe pusher

On/off switch

Visible alarm

Syringe

Syringe holder

Microbore tubing

If you anticipate your patient will need further I.V. therapy — or if the drug he's receiving can cause immediate adverse reactions — consider obtaining an order for an indwelling venipuncture device.

Injection into an existing line. To give an injection directly into the injection port of a existing line, you need the medication, a syringe with a 20G to 22G 1″ needle, and an alcohol swab. You may also need a saline-filled syringe for flushing.

To perform the procedure, follow these steps:
• Check the I.V. site for redness, tenderness, edema, or leakage.

If you detect any of these signs of complications, change the site before you administer the drug.
• If the new drug and the existing infusate are compatible, keep the infusion running. If the drug isn't compatible with the infusate but is compatible with saline solution, either change the container, piggyback a saline solution line, or use a saline-filled syringe to flush the line before injecting the drug.
• Invert the syringe and gently push the plunger to remove all air.
• Using an alcohol swab, clean the rubber cap of the injection port closest to the venipuncture device.
• Stabilize the injection port with

one hand and insert the needle through the center of the rubber cap. Don't force the insertion. If you meet resistance, position the needle at a different angle.

• Inject the drug at an even rate, as ordered. Never inject so fast that you stop the infusion or allow the drug to flow back into the tubing.

• Observe the patient for any signs of a reaction during and after the injection.

• Withdraw the needle and reestablish the desired flow rate.

Intermittent infusion

The most common and flexible method of administering I.V. drugs is intermittent infusion. By using this method over short periods at varying intervals, you can maintain therapeutic blood levels. You may deliver a small volume (25 to 250 ml) over several minutes or a few hours.

You can deliver an intermittent infusion through a piggyback line, heparin lock, or a volume-control set. (For more information, see *Intermittent infusions: Special devices,* pages 136 and 137.)

Infusion through a piggyback line.
To infuse a drug through a piggyback line, you need the medication in the piggyback minibag, piggyback tubing, an 18G to 22G 1″ needle, an alcohol swab, 1″ adhesive tape, and an extension hook for the primary container. The primary line should have a piggyback port with a backcheck valve that stops the flow from the primary line during drug infusion and returns to the primary flow after infusion. (See *Setting up a piggyback set.*)

To perform the procedure, follow these steps:

• Check the I.V. site for infiltration, phlebitis, or infection. Check the primary line for patency.

• Hang the minibag on the I.V. pole.

• Close the flow clamp on the piggyback tubing.

• Remove the covers to the minibag port and tubing spike.

• Insert the spike firmly into the minibag port.

• Secure the needle to the piggyback tubing.

• Using an alcohol swab, clean the injection port with the backcheck valve on the primary tubing.

• Remove the needle-protector cover from the piggyback tubing; make sure the needle is secure.

• Insert the needle full length into the center of the injection port.

• Secure the needle with tape.

• Lower the minibag; open the flow clamp and allow fluid from the primary container to flow up the tubing to the fill line on the drip chamber.

• Clamp the tubing; rehang the bag.

• To administer the intermittent drug, hang the primary container on the extension hook, completely open the clamp on the piggyback tubing, and set the flow rate using the drip chamber of the primary tubing.

• Because the minibag hangs higher than the primary bag, fluid flowing from it will create pressure on the backcheck valve and completely shut off fluid flow from the primary container. After the piggyback infusion is completed, the primary fluid will automatically flow again. When this happens, close the clamp on the piggyback tubing and readjust the flow rate of the primary infusion.

If the primary tubing doesn't have a backcheck valve, you must clamp the primary line; you don't need to lower the primary container. Remember to open the primary clamp when the piggyback infusion

Setting up a piggyback set

Used only for intermittent drug infusions, a piggyback set includes a secondary container (a small I.V. bag or bottle) and short tubing with a drip chamber. To use it, connect the piggyback set to a primary line via a Y-port (or piggyback port), as shown. You must use an extension hook to position the primary I.V. container below the secondary container.

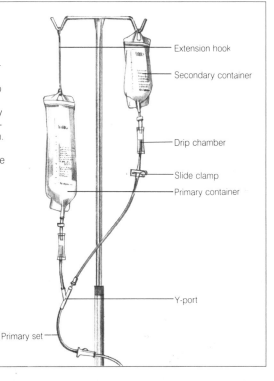

- Extension hook
- Secondary container
- Drip chamber
- Slide clamp
- Primary container
- Y-port
- Primary set

is completed. Otherwise, clots may form in the venipuncture device.

Many drugs pose a high risk of phlebitis. So be sure to check the I.V. site carefully before administering each dose. If necessary, change the site.

Heparin lock. For intermittent I.V. drug infusion with a heparin lock (also called an intermittent injection cap or intermittent infusion device), you need the drug solution in a minibag, an administration set, a 20G 1″ needle, an alcohol swab, tape, and two 3-ml syringes filled with heparin or saline flush solution (according to hospital policy) each

connected to a 20G 1″ needle.

To perform the procedure, follow these steps:
- Attach the minibag to the administration set and prime the tubing with the drug solution.
- Secure the 20G 1″ needle to the I.V. tubing adapter and prime the needle with the drug solution.
- Using an alcohol swab, clean the cap on the heparin lock.
- Stabilize the heparin lock. (See *Stabilizing a heparin lock,* page 140.)
- Insert the needle of one of the syringes containing flush solution into the center of the injection cap. Don't force it; if you feel resistance,

Stabilizing a heparin lock

Before inserting or removing a needle from a heparin lock, you must stabilize the device. To do this, grasp the lock just below the injection cap with the thumb and index finger of your non-dominant hand, as shown.

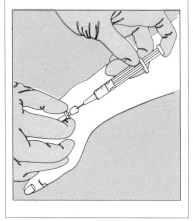

insert the needle at a different angle. Pull back on the plunger slightly and watch for blood return. If blood appears, begin to slowly inject the flush solution. If you feel any resistance or the patient complains of pain or discomfort, stop immediately because the heparin lock should be replaced.
• If you don't feel any resistance, watch for signs of infiltration as you slowly inject the flush solution. If you note signs of infiltration, replace the heparin lock; if you don't note any signs, you're ready to give the medication.
• Insert the needle attached to the administration set into the heparin lock.
• Secure the connection with tape.
• Regulate the drip rate, and infuse the medication, as ordered.
• To discontinue the infusion, close the I.V. flow clamp and withdraw the needle.
• Clean the injection cap and again flush the heparin lock.

Remember, before accessing the lock, check the I.V. site carefully and change it if necessary.

Access the intermittent cap with a needle of the appropriate gauge and length. A 20G needle is large enough that it won't break and small enough that it won't cause leaks. A 1″ needle allows a secure connection without the risk of puncturing the catheter or tubing.

When the injection cap serves as a heparin lock, stabilize the cap while accessing and removing the I.V. tubing and needle to prevent stress at the insertion site. Stress increases the risks of phlebitis and catheter dislodgment.

You must be present when the infusion runs out so you can disconnect the tubing and flush the device. Otherwise clots will form in the heparin lock.

Flush the device after each use and when it's not in use with the type and volume of solution recommended by hospital policy. The flush solution may be saline or diluted heparin. Flushing may be required every 6 to 24 hours.

You also need to follow your hospital's policy for tubing changes. If you have to reconnect used tubing, be sure the tubing needle-adapter hasn't been contaminated. And always use a sterile needle.

You can also give medications by direct injection through a heparin lock. In this case, flush the heparin lock, inject the medication as ordered, and flush the heparin lock again.

Volume-control set. You can use a volume-control set as either a primary or secondary line. Either way, remember these sets are expensive and pose a high risk of contamination. So make sure you closely follow your hospital's policies concerning their use.

When using a volume-control set as a primary line, you need the I.V. solution, medication in a syringe with a 20G 1″ needle, alcohol swabs, and a label.

When using a volume-control set as a secondary line, you need the I.V. solution, 20G 1″ needle, adhesive tape (for piggybacking), medication in a syringe with a 20G 1″ needle, alcohol swabs, and a label.

To perform the procedure, follow these steps:
● Check the I.V. line for patency and the I.V. site for infiltration, phlebitis, and infection.
● If you're using the volume-control set as a primary line, prime the tubing with the I.V. solution. Then insert the adapter of the set into the catheter or needle hub of the venipuncture device. If you're using the volume-control set as a secondary line, attach the 20G 1″ needle to the adapter on the set and prime the tubing and needle with the I.V. solution. Then wipe the injection site on the primary tubing with an alcohol swab, insert the needle into the injection port, and tape the connection.
● To add medication to the chamber, wipe the injection port on the volume-control set with an alcohol swab and inject the medication. (See *Adding medication to a volume-control set*.)
● Place a label on the chamber indicating the drug, dose, time, and date. Don't write directly on the chamber with ink (the plastic will absorb the ink). Also, don't place the label over the numbers of the chamber.
● Open the upper clamp; fill the

Adding medication to a volume-control set

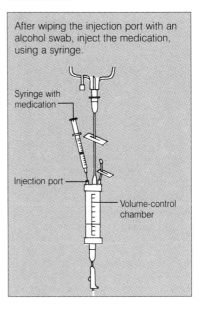

After wiping the injection port with an alcohol swab, inject the medication, using a syringe.

Syringe with medication

Injection port

Volume-control chamber

fluid chamber with the prescribed amount of solution to dilute the medication. Close the clamp. Gently rotate the chamber to mix the medication and the solution.
● If you're using the volume-control set as a secondary line, either stop the primary infusion, or set a low drip rate so the line will be open when the secondary infusion is completed.
● Open the lower clamp of the volume-control set, and adjust the drip rate as ordered.
● After the infusion is completed and if the patient can tolerate the extra fluid, open the upper clamp and let 10 ml of I.V. solution flow into the chamber and through the tubing to flush it and deliver all the medication to the patient.
● If you're using the volume-control set as a secondary line, close the

lower clamp and reset the flow rate on the primary line. If you're using the set as a primary line, close the lower clamp, refill the chamber to the prescribed amount of primary solution, and restart the infusion.

Instead of using the volume-control set as a primary line, you can mix the medication in the primary solution. Then use the volume-control chamber to closely regulate the amount of fluid and drug dosage the patient receives.

If you're using a volume-control set that has a membrane for intermittent drug administration, fill the chamber with fluid before adding the medication. This prevents the membrane from becoming sticky and difficult to operate. All manufacturers give specific instructions for priming volume-control sets, but a set with a membrane can be difficult to prime.

An easy way to remember how to prime this set is to fill the chamber with at least 20 ml of fluid, then think OSCAR: **O**pen the flow-regulating clamp; **S**queeze and hold the drip chamber; **C**lose the regulating clamp directly below the drip chamber; **A**nd **R**elease the drip chamber.

The infusion will stop when the fluid chamber is empty. If the set doesn't have a membrane or shut-off valve, refill the fluid chamber quickly to prevent an infusion of air.

Continuous infusion

Given through a peripheral or central venous line, a continuous infusion of medication allows you to carefully regulate drug delivery over a prolonged period. Sometimes, before you start a continuous infusion, you'll give a loading dose to achieve peak serum levels quickly.

A continuous infusion enhances the effectiveness of some drugs such as lidocaine and heparin, which are often regulated with an I.V. pump or controller.

Infusion through a primary line.
When administering a continuous infusion through a primary line, you need the prescribed medication in I.V. solution, an administration set, and gloves. You may also need an infusion pump or controller. If so, make sure you have the correct administration set for the pump or controller.

To perform the procedure, follow these steps:
• Make sure the I.V. solution container is labeled with the name and dosage of the medication.
• Attach the administration set to the solution container and prime the tubing with the I.V. solution. Attach the administration set to the pump or controller, if appropriate.
• If necessary, perform or assist with the venipuncture.
• To begin the infusion, put on gloves and remove the protective cap at the end of the administration set. Then attach the set to the venipuncture device.
• Begin the infusion and regulate the flow to the ordered rate.
• Frequently monitor the patient and the flow rate.
• When the infusion is completed, hang another solution, as ordered. If the patient will be receiving only intermittent I.V. medications, convert the device into a heparin lock.

Maintain accurate intake and output records and be alert for excessive fluid retention and fluid overload. When a patient receives small amounts hourly, his total daily volume can be excessive without the problem being obvious.

Remember too that giving a large volume of fluid can change a patient's electrolyte levels. Be sure to check the patient's laboratory results to make sure his electrolyte levels stay within normal limits.

Check the flow rate at regular intervals to ensure delivery of the medication as ordered. Also check I.V. sites frequently for signs of complications. If you note tenderness, redness, swelling, or leakage, discontinue the infusion and treat the site according to hospital policy. Restart the infusion in another vein.

Infusion through a secondary line. To give a continuous infusion through a secondary line, you need the prescribed medication in I.V. solution, an administration set, 20G 1″ needle, alcohol swabs, and 1″ adhesive tape. You may also need an infusion pump or controller. If so, make sure you have the correct administration set for the pump or controller.

To perform the procedure, follow these steps:
• Attach the administration set to the solution container and prime the tubing with the I.V. solution. If appropriate, attach the administration set to the pump or controller.
• Secure the 20G 1″ needle to the administration set and prime the needle with the I.V. solution.
• Using adhesive tape, place labels with the name of the drug under the drip chamber and at the end of the tubing.
• Clean the injection port on the primary tubing with an alcohol swab.
• Insert the needle, full length, into the center of the injection port. Secure the needle with tape.
• Regulate the drip rate of the secondary solution and adjust the rate of the primary solution.
• Frequently monitor the patient and the infusion rate.
• When the secondary infusion is completed, remove the needle from the injection port. Adjust the flow rate of the primary solution.

Check for an immediate, visible incompatibility. Especially when using multiple lines, make sure all drugs are compatible.

To prevent confusion when using multiple secondary lines, don't let them become tangled. Tag the lines below the drip chamber and at the connection site to the primary line. This clearly identifies the source and tubing connection for each drug.

If hospital policy permits, use a pump to achieve more accurate dosage control. Put a time strip on the secondary container to help monitor the administration rate.

Maintain a secure, patent venipuncture device. To avoid interrupting drug therapy when you change the I.V. site, establish the new site before disconnecting the old one. Also firmly stabilize the connection to the primary tubing with tape or a locking device to prevent a broken needle or dislodgment.

If attaching the secondary line to the primary line with a needle in an injection port, use a 20G 1″ needle. A larger gauge needle may cause leaks. A longer needle may pierce the tubing. A needleless system eliminates these concerns.

Patient-controlled analgesia
An alternative administration method, PCA therapy allows your patient to control I.V. delivery of an analgesic (usually morphine) and maintain therapeutic serum levels. He uses a specialized infusion device with a timing unit that delivers a dose of an analgesic at a controlled volume. (See *Understanding PCA devices*, page 144.)

The doctor's order should include:
• a loading dose, which is given by I.V. push at the start of PCA therapy

Understanding PCA devices

A patient-controlled analgesia (PCA) device allows your patient to receive an analgesic by pushing a button. A timing unit prevents him from accidentally overdosing by imposing a lock-out time between doses—usually 6 to 10 minutes. During this interval, the patient won't receive any analgesic despite pushing the button.

PCA devices come in several types; below are two of the more common ones.

P.C.A. PUMP WITH CALL-BUTTON

With this reusable, battery-operated PCA pump, the patient triggers drug delivery by pressing a button attached to a cord.

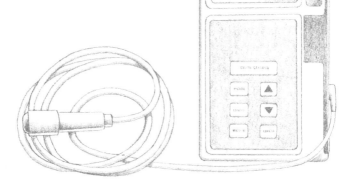

P.C.A. DEVICE WITH WRISTBAND

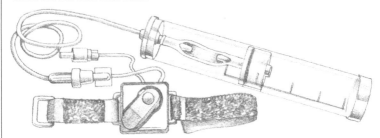

This disposable, mechanically operated PCA device contains an infusor and a unit that's worn like a wristwatch. The patient pushes a button on the device to receive the analgesic. No more than 0.5 ml of solution can be delivered in 6 minutes.

(frequently 25 mg meperidine [Demerol] or 2 mg morphine)
- a lock-out interval, during which the PCA device can't be activated (usually 6 to 10 minutes)
- the maintenance dose
- the amount the patient will receive when he activates the device (frequently 10 mg Demerol or 1 mg morphine)
- the maximum amount the patient can receive within a specified time (if an adjustable device is used).

Indications and advantages. Indicated for patients who need parenteral analgesia, PCA therapy is commonly given to trauma patients postoperatively. It's also being administered to patients with chronic diseases — particularly those with terminal cancer.

To receive PCA therapy, a patient must be mentally alert, able to understand and comply with instructions and procedures, and have no history of an allergy to the analgesic. Patients not eligible for therapy include those who have a limited respiratory reserve, a history of drug abuse or chronic sedative or tranquilizer use, or a psychiatric disorder.

PCA therapy eliminates the need for I.M. analgesics. It also provides individualized pain relief, with each patient receiving the appropriate dosage for his size and pain tolerance. Plus, it gives the patient a sense of control over his pain. This therapy also allows the patient to sleep at night, while minimizing daytime drowsiness. Finally, patients receiving PCA therapy use less narcotics for pain relief than other patients.

Adverse effects. Because the primary adverse effect of analgesics is respiratory depression, you must routinely monitor your patient's respiratory rate. Also, check for infiltration into the subcutaneous tissues and for catheter occlusion, which may cause the drug to back up in the primary I.V. tubing. If the analgesic makes your patient nauseated, he may need an antinausea drug.

Starting therapy. Before your patient starts using the PCA device, teach him how it works. Then have him practice with a sample PCA device. Make it clear that he shouldn't expect complete pain relief. Explain that he should take enough analgesic to relieve acute pain but not so much that he becomes sleepy.

During therapy, you'll need to monitor and record the amount of analgesic infused, the patient's respiratory rate, and his assessment of the pain relief. If he doesn't feel that his pain has been sufficiently relieved, notify the doctor, who may increase the dosage.

Maintaining therapy

When giving I.V. medications to a pediatric or elderly patient, you'll need to be aware of some special considerations. Also, if you're caring for a patient who'll continue I.V. medication therapy at home, you'll have to teach him to do so. And when caring for any patient receiving I.V. medication therapy, you must know how to recognize and treat certain complications.

Patients with special needs
Certain patients — particularly pediatric, elderly, and home care patients — have special needs during I.V. medication therapy. Some tips

Using the retrograde system

To use this method, add a segment of coiled low-volume tubing with a three-way stopcock at each end to the primary I.V. tubing, as shown. Connect an empty syringe (the displacement syringe) to the stopcock closer to the I.V. container. Then connect a syringe containing the diluted drug (medication syringe) to the stopcock closer to the patient. Turn the distal stopcock off to the I.V. container and the proximal stopcock off to the patient.

As you inject the drug it will flow away from the patient (in a retrograde direction) into the coiled low-volume tubing. This forces an equal volume of fluid into the displacement syringe.

Next, turn both stopcocks off to the syringes. The diluted drug in the low-volume tubing will now be infused without increasing the patient's fluid intake.

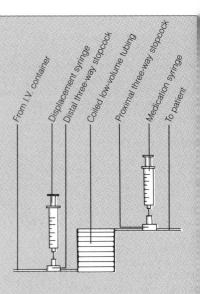

and techniques you'll use when caring for these patients are covered in this section.

Pediatric patients. Neonates and infants have precise fluid requirements, and small children can't tolerate the large amount of fluid recommended for diluting many drugs. Because the drug dosage is based on the child's weight, each patient will have a different normal dosage. Also, because of the small drug volume and slow delivery, you must make sure that no drug remains in the I.V. tubing before you change it.

The most common method of giving I.V. drugs to pediatric patients is intermittent infusion, using a volume-control set. When setting up the equipment for a pediatric

patient, keep flow-control clamps out of his reach. Also, use tamper-proof pumps so he can't change the rate.

In many cases, the venipuncture device will stay in place longer than it would for an adult. So you must be especially careful to protect the I.V. site from stress and use aseptic technique whenever you're administering I.V. medications.

• *Retrograde administration.* One way of overcoming the problem of infants' precise fluid requirements is retrograde administration. This administration method allows you to give an I.V. antibiotic over a 30-minute period without increasing fluid volume. (See *Using the retrograde system.*)

For this method, you need only one tubing to administer all I.V.

luids and medications. And you don't have to change the primary flow rate to administer I.V. drugs.

Disadvantages include unpredictable drug delivery — particularly with flow rates of less than 5 ml/hour. The low-volume tubing must be able to hold the entire diluted drug volume. If any is displaced into the syringe, it will be discarded. Also, the drug must be diluted in a volume equal to half the ml/hour rate of the primary infusion to allow for a 30-minute drug infusion. So, if the primary rate is changed, the diluted drug volume must be changed, too.

• *Syringe pump.* You'll find that a syringe pump is especially useful for giving intermittent I.V. medications to pediatric patients. The reason: It gives you the greatest control for small-volume infusions.

Be sure the pump you use is tamperproof and has a built-in guard against uncontrolled flow rates and an alarm sensitive to low-pressure occlusion. It should operate accurately with syringe sizes from 1 to 60 ml using low-volume tubing.

• *Intraosseous infusion.* When venous access can't be established in an emergency, an alternative method of drug delivery, intraosseous infusion, may be used. Typically performed by emergency personnel, intraosseous infusion is a simple, quick, and relatively safe method for short-term administration of drugs. The drugs may be given by continuous or intermittent infusion or by direct injection just as quickly and effectively as with the I.V. route. However, intraosseous infusion should be used only until venous access can be established.

Elderly patients. When administering an I.V. analgesic to an elderly patient, monitor him for respiratory depression. When giving a drug that can cause renal toxicity, monitor the patient closely for this complication. Remember, many elderly patients have decreased pulmonary and renal functions.

Because many elderly patients have fragile veins, they're prone to infiltration and phlebitis. So carefully assess the I.V. site for signs and symptoms of these complications. If necessary, restart the infusion before you administer a drug by any method.

Many I.V. drugs are particularly irritating to fragile veins, so you may have to dilute a drug in a larger volume than you normally would. Remember though, elderly patients are prone to fluid overload. Keep accurate intake and output records, and include all fluids given for I.V. drug administration.

Home care patients. If your patient will be receiving I.V. medications at home, you'll usually begin teaching him or his home caregiver while he's in the hospital. As you teach, be sure to give the patient written instructions for each step of the procedure. Make sure he knows how to prevent and recognize complications of therapy. He also must know what to do when a complication does occur.

• *Administering antibiotics.* With home care patients, I.V. antibiotics are usually given intermittently through a heparin lock. Patients who must leave their homes to work may be supplied with a simple-to-use, small-volume infusion device that automatically delivers drug solutions at a preset rate. (See *I.V. infusion with a spring-operated syringe,* page 148.)

Explain to the patient that a pharmacist at the home care agency or pharmacy service will mix the

I.V. infusion with a spring-operated syringe

When an ambulatory patient needs infusions of I.V. medication, one option is a spring-operated syringe, such as ADFuse, which consists of a disposable 60-ml syringe with small-volume extension tubing. The device automatically infuses 1.25 ml/minute with pressure from the built-in spring. The medication will be infused regardless of the position of the syringe.

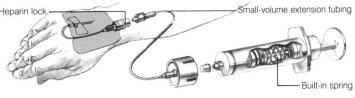

Heparin lock ⎯⎯⎯⎯⎯⎯⎯⎯⎯⎯⎯⎯⎯⎯⎯ Small-volume extension tubing

Built-in spring

drug solutions. Also, explain that a home care nurse will routinely change the I.V. site.

Teach the patient to check the I.V. site for complications before each dose. He should report any problems before administering the drug.

Be sure your patient understands the need for aseptic technique. Show him how to insert the needle without contaminating it. Also, teach him about the possible adverse effects of the particular drug he'll be receiving. Typically, the first dose will be given while he's still hospitalized to minimize the risk of adverse effects at home.

• *Administering pain medication.* Usually, long-term I.V. pain therapy is given by continuous infusion, using a central venous catheter connected to an external or an implanted pump. Either pump may be able to deliver bolus injections.

A continuous infusion will also be used for short-term therapy. But the drug solution will be delivered by a peripheral I.V. line connected to a pump that may or may not be able to deliver bolus injections.

A patient receiving I.V. pain medication through a central catheter with an external pump may not be able to perform the required procedures. So a home caregiver or a private-duty nurse must perform them. If you're teaching the home caregiver, be sure to discuss the container, tubing, and dressing changes. Make sure he can operate and troubleshoot the pump. If the patient will need bolus injections, teach the home caregiver how to monitor the patient for adverse effects of the drug.

A patient receiving I.V. pain medication through an implanted pump won't need special care between pump refills, which are done by a doctor or home care nurse. The patient rarely needs a bolus.

Typically, short-term I.V. pain control through a peripheral infusion will be used for a patient close to death. In such cases, you should teach the caregiver to change containers, operate the pump, monitor the I.V. site, check for adverse drug reactions, and if necessary, deliver bolus injections. The home care nurse will usually change the venipuncture device and tubing.

Complications

To protect any patient receiving I.V. medication therapy, watch for signs and symptoms of serious complications — hypersensitivity, extravasation, phlebitis, and infection.

Hypersensitivity. Before you administer a drug, ask the patient if he has any allergies, including ones to food or pollen. Also, ask if he has a family history of allergies. Patients with a personal or family history of allergies are more likely to develop a drug hypersensitivity.

If your patient is an infant under 3 months old, be sure to ask about the mother's allergy history because maternal antibodies may still be present. Hypersensitivity, however, is far less common in infants and children than in adults.

After giving an I.V. drug, stay with the patient for 5 to 10 minutes to detect signs and symptoms of hypersensitivity — sudden fever, joint swelling, rash, hives, bronchospasm, and wheezing. If he's receiving the drug for the first time, keep checking him every 5 to 10 minutes. Otherwise, check every 30 minutes for a few hours.

At the first sign of hypersensitivity, discontinue the drug infusion and notify the doctor. Remember, immediate severe reactions are life-threatening. If necessary, assist with emergency treatment.

Extravasation. This complication often stems from improper placement or dislodgment of the catheter. In elderly patients, extravasation may occur because the veins are thin and fragile.

The risk of extravasation increases when the venipuncture device remains in the vein for more than 2 days or when the tip is positioned near a flexion area. In these cases, patient movement may cause the venipuncture device to retract from the vein.

If only a small amount of an isotonic solution or nonirritating drug extravasates, the patient will usually experience only mild discomfort. You can treat him with routine comfort measures, such as warm soaks. But extravasation of vesicant drugs — such as various antineoplastic drugs and sympathomimetics — can produce severe local tissue damage. Such damage not only causes discomfort but may also delay healing, produce infection and disfigurement, and lead to loss of function and possibly amputation.

If you suspect extravasation, stop the I.V. infusion at once and elevate the patient's arm. Subsequent treatment varies, depending on the drug and the hospital's policy. (See *Preventing and treating extravasation,* page 150, and *Antidotes for vesicant extravasation,* page 151.)

• *Assessment misconceptions.* Frequently, nurses test for blood return to determine if extravasation is occurring. But the absence of a blood return doesn't always indicate extravasation. If you're using a small needle in a small vein or in one with low venous pressure, blood return may not be possible. Nor will it be possible if the tip of the venipuncture device is pressed against the vein wall.

Another common misconception is that extravasation always causes a hard lump. When the needle tip is completely out of the vein wall, a lump may form. But if fluid leaks out of the vein slowly (as it may when the needle tip partially pierces the vein wall), extravasation may just produce a flat, diffuse swelling. Keep in mind, too, that your

(Text continues on page 152.)

COMPLICATIONS

Preventing and treating extravasation

Extravasation—the infiltration of a drug into the surrounding tissue—can occur when a vein is punctured or when there's leakage around an I.V. site. If vesicant (blistering) drugs or fluids extravasate, severe local tissue damage often results.

Prevention

To prevent extravasation when you're giving vesicants, adhere strictly to proper administration techniques and follow these guidelines:
• Don't use an existing I.V. line unless its patency is assured. Perform a new venipuncture to ensure correct needle placement and vein patency.
• Select the site carefully. Use a distal vein that allows successive proximal venipunctures. To avoid tendon and nerve damage from possible extravasation, avoid using the dorsum of the hand. Also, avoid the wrist and digits (they're hard to immobilize) and areas previously damaged or with compromised circulation.
• If you need to probe for a vein, you may cause trauma. Stop and begin again at another site.
• Start the infusion with dextrose 5% in water (D₅W) or saline solution.
• Check for extravasation before giving the medication. Apply a tourniquet above the needle to occlude the vein; then see if the flow continues. If the flow stops, the solution isn't infiltrating. Another method you can use is to lower the I.V. container and watch for blood backflow. This is less reliable because the needle may have punctured the opposite vein wall but still be resting partially in the vein. Flush the needle to ensure patency. If swelling occurs at the I.V. site, the solution is infiltrating.
• Give drugs by slow I.V. push through a free-flowing I.V. line or by small-volume infusion (50 to 100 ml).
• Give vesicants last when multiple drugs are ordered. If possible, avoid using an infusion pump to administer vesicants. A pump will continue the infusion if infiltration occurs.
• During administration, observe the infusion site for erythema or infiltration. Tell your patient to report any burning, stinging, pain, pruritus, or temperature changes.
• Use a transparent semipermeable dressing to allow inspection of the I.V. site.
• After drug administration, instill several milliliters of D₅W or saline solution to flush the drug from the vein and to preclude drug leakage when the needle is removed.

Treatment

If extravasation occurs, emergency treatment is required. Follow your hospital's protocol. Essential steps should include the following:
• Stop the I.V. flow and remove the I.V. line, unless you need the needle to infiltrate the antidote.
• Estimate the amount of extravasated solution and notify the doctor.
• Instill the appropriate antidote according to hospital protocol.
• Elevate the extremity.
• Record the extravasation site, the patient's symptoms, the estimated amount of infiltrated solution, and the treatment. Also record the time you notified the doctor and his name. Continue documenting the appearance of the site and associated symptoms.
• Following hospital protocol, apply either ice packs or warm compresses to the affected area.
• If skin breakdown occurs, apply silver sulfadiazine cream and gauze dressings or wet-to-dry povidone-iodine dressings, as ordered.
  If severe debridement occurs, your patient may need plastic surgery and physical therapy.

OMPLICATIONS

Antidotes for vesicant extravasation

Usually, you'll give an antidote for vesicant extravasation in one of two ways—either by instilling it through an existing I.V. line to infiltrate the area or by injecting small amounts subcutaneously in a circle around the infiltrated area, using a 1-ml syringe. With the latter method, you should change needles before each injection.

The following chart lists common antidotes you may administer. Some will be used in combination with others.

ANTIDOTE	DOSE	EXTRAVASATED DRUG
Ascorbic acid injection	50 mg	dactinomycin
Hyaluronidase 15 units/ml Mix a 150-unit vial with 1 ml normal saline solution for injection. Withdraw 0.1 ml and dilute with 0.9 ml normal saline solution to get 15 units/ml.	0.2 ml × five subcutaneous injections around site	aminophylline calcium solutions contrast media dextrose solutions (concentrations of 10% or more) nafcillin potassium solutions total parenteral nutrition solutions vinblastine vincristine vindesine
Hydrocortisone sodium succinate 100 mg/ml Usually followed by topical application of hydrocortisone cream 1%.	50 to 200 mg (25 to 50 mg/ml of extravasate)	doxorubicin vincristine
Phentolamine Dilute 5 to 10 mg with 10 ml of normal saline solution for injection.	5 to 10 mg	dobutamine dopamine epinephrine metaraminol bitartrate norepinephrine
Sodium bicarbonate 8.4%	5 ml	carmustine daunorubicin doxorubicin vinblastine vincristine
Sodium edetate	150 mg	plicamycin
Sodium thiosulfate 10% Dilute 4 ml with 6 ml sterile water for injection.	10 ml	dactinomycin mechlorethamine mitomycin

COMPLICATIONS

Detecting phlebitis

If you detect postinfusion phlebitis early, it can be treated effectively. If undetected, however, phlebitis can cause local infection, severe discomfort, and sepsis.

Here's a brief explanation of how the signs and symptoms of phlebitis develop. As platelets aggregate at the damage site, a thrombus begins to form and histamine, bradykinin, and serotonin are released. The increased blood flow to the injury site and the thrombus formation at the vein wall cause redness, tenderness, and slight edema.

If you don't remove the venipuncture device at this stage, the vein wall becomes hard and tender and may develop a red streak 2″ to 6″ (5 to 15 cm) long. Left untreated, phlebitis may produce exudate at the I.V. site, accompanied by elevated WBC count and fever. It can also produce pain at the I.V. site, but the lack of pain doesn't eliminate the possibility of phlebitis.

You classify the degree of phlebitis as follows:

1+ Pain with no erythema, swelling, induration, or palpable venous cord.

2+ Pain, some erythema, some swelling, or both; absence of induration or a palpable venous cord.

3+ Pain, erythema, swelling with induration or a palpable venous cord less than 3″ (7.5 cm) above site.

4+ Pain, erythema, swelling, induration, and a palpable venous cord greater than 3″ above site.

patient may not always experience coldness or discomfort with extravasation. He may feel cold if extravasation occurs during rapid administration of a medication. But rarely will a patient feel cold from extravasation during a slow infusion.

Phlebitis. Postinfusion phlebitis, a common complication of I.V. therapy, is often associated with drugs or solutions that have a low pH or high osmolarity. Other contributing factors include vein trauma during insertion, use of too small a vein or too large an insertion device, and prolonged use of the same I.V. site.

More common after continuous infusions, phlebitis can follow any infusion — or even an injection of a single drug. Typically, it develops 2 to 3 days after the vein is exposed to the drug or solution. Phlebitis develops more rapidly in distal veins than in the larger veins close to the heart.

Drugs given by direct injection generally don't cause phlebitis when administered at the correct dilution and rate. However, phenytoin and diazepam, which are frequently given by this method, can produce phlebitis after one or more injections at the same I.V. site.

When piggybacked, certain irritating I.V. drugs are likely to cause phlebitis. These include erythromycin, tetracycline, nafcillin sodium, vancomycin, and amphotericin B. Adding 250 to 1,000 ml of diluent reduces the risk of irritation. But you still should change the I.V. site every 24 to 48 hours. Large doses potassium chloride (40 mEq/liter or more), amino acids, dextrose solutions (10% or more), and multivitamins can also cause phlebitis.

Phlebitis can result too from motion and pressure of the venipuncture device. Also, particles in drugs and I.V. solutions can produce phlebitis. You can reduce the risk of phlebitis from this cause by using filter needles and I.V. filters.

• *Detection and prevention.* To detect phlebitis, inspect the I.V. site several times daily. Use a transparent semipermeable dressing or minimal adhesive tape so you can see the skin distal to the tip of the venipuncture device. At the first sign of redness or tenderness, move the venipuncture device to another site, preferably on the opposite arm. (See *Detecting phlebitis.*) To ease your patient's discomfort, apply warm packs or soak the arm in warm water.

To help prevent phlebitis, the pharmacist can alter drug osmolarity and pH. But the main responsibility for prevention rests with you. These measures will help you avoid phlebitis:
• Use proper venipuncture technique.
• Dilute drugs correctly.
• Monitor administration rates.
• Observe the I.V. site frequently.
• Change the injection site regularly.

Infection. A patient receiving I.V. medication therapy may develop a local infection at the I.V. site. So monitor your patient for signs and symptoms such as extreme redness or discharge at the site.

Also, keep in mind that you're at risk for serious infection. If your patient has the hepatitis B virus or human immunodeficiency virus (HIV), it can be transmitted from him to those caring for him. To protect yourself, follow the precautions for handling blood and body fluids recommended by the CDC.

Remember to treat all patients as potentially infected with HIV and take appropriate precautions. Also, if you'll be administering I.V. drugs and solutions, you should receive the hepatitis B vaccine (if you don't already have hepatitis B antibodies.) This vaccine is effective for at least 5 years and produces antibodies in 95% of those vaccinated.

Suggested readings

Akahoshi, M.P., et al. "Patient Controlled Analgesia via Intrathecal Catheter in Outpatient Oncology Patients," *Journal of Intravenous Nursing* 11(5):289-92, September/October 1988.

Brown, J.M. "Innovative Antibiotic Therapy at Home," *Journal of Intravenous Nursing* 11(6):397-401, November/December 1988.

Mellema, S.J., and Poniatowski, B.C. "Geriatric I.V. Therapy," *Journal of Intravenous Nursing* 11(1):56-61, January/February 1988.

Physician's Desk Reference (PDR), 44th ed. Oradell, N.J.: Medical Economics Company, 1990.

Plumer, A.L. *Principles and Practice of Intravenous Therapy,* 4th ed. Boston: Little, Brown & Co., 1987.

Turco, S., and King, R. *Sterile Dosage Forms,* 3rd ed. Philadelphia: Lea & Febiger, 1987.

Wheeler, G.A. "Pediatric Intraosseous Infusion: An Old Technique in Modern Health Care Technology," *Journal of Intravenous Nursing* 12(6):371-76, November/December 1989.

6
TRANSFUSION

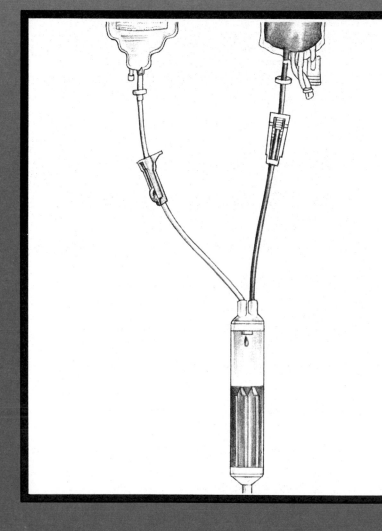

Transfusion therapy can restore blood volume or correct deficiencies in the blood's oxygen-carrying capacity or coagulation components. Depending on your patient's condition, you may administer a transfusion through a peripheral I.V. line or a central venous (CV) line. Typically, a peripheral I.V. line delivers limited transfusions. In contrast, a CV line delivers massive transfusions.

This chapter will help you sharpen your transfusion skills by explaining the principles and procedures you need to know. In the first section, you'll review the indications for transfusion, as well as the basic composition and physiology of blood. The next section tells you how to transfuse whole blood, cellular components, plasma, and plasma fractions. This section includes a brief discussion of hemapheresis and autotransfusion — two specialized means of administering blood. In the last section of the chapter, you'll review special considerations for pediatric, elderly, and home care patients. Plus, you'll find valuable information on how to recognize and treat the common complications of transfusion.

Basic concepts

A doctor may order a transfusion for a patient when illness or injury decreases the blood's volume, oxygen-carrying capacity, or coagulation components. A decrease in blood volume can result from hemorrhage, trauma, or burns, while depleted oxygen-carrying capacity generally stems from respiratory disorders, carbon monoxide poisoning, absolute anemia, or sickle cell disease. Coagulation component deficiency can result from hemorrhage, hepatic failure, bone marrow suppression, thrombocytopenia, medication- and disease-induced qualitative coagulopathies, or vitamin K deficiency.

Many states allow RNs (but not LPNs) to administer blood and blood components. In some states, however, LPNs may regulate transfusion flow rates, observe patients for reactions, discontinue transfusions, and document the procedures.

When transfusing blood, remember to protect yourself from exposure to transmittable diseases, such as viral hepatitis and acquired immunodeficiency syndrome (AIDS). The Centers for Disease Control guidelines recommend wearing gloves, a mask, and a gown when transfusing blood, in case the blood spills or sprays.

Before starting a transfusion, always consider its therapeutic value and the patient's expected outcome. Even a lifesaving transfusion can result in potentially life-threatening complications, such as a hemolytic reaction. When the transfusion of blood components is contraindicated, fluid infusions can restore decreased blood volume.

Blood composition and physiology

Blood contains two basic components: cellular (or formed) elements and plasma. Consisting of erythrocytes (red blood cells [RBCs]), leukocytes (white blood cells [WBCs]), and thrombocytes (platelets), the cellular elements make up about 45% of blood volume. Plasma, the liquid component, makes up about 55% of blood volume. It consists of water (serum) and protein (albumin, globulin, and fibrinogen), as well as lipids, electrolytes, vitamins, carbohydrates, nonprotein nitrogen compounds, bilirubin, and gases.

Current techniques allow the separation of freshly donated whole blood into its component fractions: RBCs, plasma, platelets, granulocytes, immune globulin, albumin, and plasma protein. These components can correct specific hematologic deficiencies, making it unnecessary to transfuse whole blood. Generally, only a patient who's lost massive quantities of blood within a short time receives a whole blood transfusion.

Antigens and antibodies. Blood also contains two other major components: antigens and antibodies. Existing on the surfaces of blood cells, antigens can initiate an immune response. A particular antigen also can induce the formation of a corresponding antibody when given to a person who doesn't normally have the antigen. An antibody is an immunoglobulin molecule synthesized in response to a specific antigen. The body inherits the established major antigens, such as those in the ABO system and the Rh-Hr system. Exogenous sources, such as blood transfusions, introduce other antigens into the body.

• *Compatibility tests.* Before a transfusion, various laboratory tests are used to identify naturally occurring or acquired antigens and antibodies in both the recipient and the donor. These tests detect any incompatibilities between recipient and donor blood that could produce a transfusion reaction. The most important tests include ABO blood typing, Rh typing, cross matching, the direct antiglobulin test, and the antibody screening test. (The donor's blood will also be screened for hepatitis B, syphilis, AIDS, and cytomegalovirus [CMV].)

Keep in mind that the tests for recipient-donor compatibility aren't foolproof. A transfusion reaction can occur despite the use of compatible blood. In such cases, other tests for antibodies (such as leukoagglutinins) can help identify the cause and prevent further reactions.

• *ABO blood group.* The ABO system classifies human RBCs as either A, B, AB, or O. The system also includes two naturally occurring antibodies: anti-A and anti-B, one, both, or neither of which may be found in the plasma. (See *Reviewing blood type compatibility.*)

Because group O blood lacks both A and B antigens, you can transfuse it in limited amounts in an emergency to any patient — regardless of his blood type — with little risk of agglutination. For this reason, people with group O blood are called universal donors. (However, the transfusion should be given as packed RBCs, from which 80% of the plasma has been removed.) A person with AB blood has neither anti-A nor anti-B antibodies, so he can receive A, B, or O blood (packed RBCs), making him a universal recipient.

A typing and cross matching test establishes the compatibility of the donor and recipient blood and minimizes the risk of a hemolytic reaction — the greatest danger with blood transfusions. Such a reaction occurs when the donor and recipient blood types are mismatched — for instance, when blood containing anti-A antibodies mixes with blood containing B antigens. When mismatching occurs, the antibodies attach to the surfaces of the recipient's RBCs, causing the cells to clump together. Eventually, these clumped cells can plug small blood vessels.

This antibody-antigen reaction

Reviewing blood type compatibility

Precise blood typing and cross matching can prevent the transfusion of incompatible blood, which can be fatal. Usually, typing the recipient's blood and cross matching it with available donor blood takes less than 1 hour.

Agglutinogen (antigen in red blood cells [RBCs]) and agglutinin (antibody in plasma) distinguish the four ABO blood groups. This chart shows you ABO compatibility at a glance from the perspective of the recipient and the donor.

Blood group	Antibodies present in plasma	Compatible RBCs	Compatible plasma
RECIPIENT			
O	Anti-A and Anti-B	O	O, A, B, AB
A	Anti-B	A, O	A, AB
B	Anti-A	B, O	B, AB
AB	Neither Anti-A nor Anti-B	AB, A, B, O	AB
DONOR			
O	Anti-A and Anti-B	O, A, B, AB	O
A	Anti-B	A, AB	A, O
B	Anti-A	B, AB	B, O
AB	Neither Anti-A nor Anti-B	AB	AB, A, B, O

activates the body's complement system — a group of enzymatic proteins that promotes and accelerates RBC hemolysis and phagocytosis by the reticuloendothelial cells. RBC hemolysis releases free hemoglobin into the bloodstream, which can damage the renal tubules and lead to renal failure and death.

● *Rh blood group.* Another major blood antigen system, the Rhesus (Rh) system, has two groups: Rh negative and Rh positive. Rh-positive blood has the D antigen; Rh-negative blood does not. If a person with Rh-negative blood receives Rh-positive blood, $Rh_o(D)$ positive immunization will occur, resulting in RBC hemolysis.

In the United States, about 85% of Whites and an even higher percentage of Blacks, Native Americans, and Asians have Rh-positive blood. The rest of the population has Rh-negative blood.

Because of its high immunogenicity, Rh antigen may be more likely to stimulate antibody formation than other known antigens. A person with Rh-positive blood doesn't carry anti-Rh antibodies in his serum because they would destroy his RBCs. A person with Rh-negative blood, however, develops anti-Rh antibodies following exposure to Rh-positive blood either by transfusion or pregnancy. Usually, a transfusion reaction doesn't occur after the initial exposure to Rh-positive blood because anti-Rh antibodies develop slowly, causing the transfusion recipient to become sensitized to the Rh antigen. Subsequent exposure to Rh-positive blood triggers a transfusion reaction and hemolysis, as in hemolytic disease of the newborn.

An important variant in the Rh system is the D^u subantigen, which appears somewhat less immunogenic than $Rh_o(D)$. The D^u antigen may not trigger antibody production in those who lack it. However, all prospective donors must be screened for this antigen, more commonly found in blacks than in whites. Individuals whose blood contains the D^u antigen are considered Rh-positive donors — but Rh-negative recipients. This precaution protects recipients with a D^u variant because their blood may not be serologically distinguishable from D^u blood.

Other clinically significant Rh antigens, such as Rh2 (C, rh'), Rh3 (E, rh"), Rh4 (c, hr'), and Rh5 (e, hr"), appear much less immunogenic and aren't as likely to produce an antibody reaction. Tests for these antigens, done only in special cases, establish paternity, analyze family patterns, and distinguish between heterozygous and homozygous Rh-positive factors.

• *HLA blood group.* Although they exist on the surfaces of all nucleated cells, human leukocyte antigens (HLAs) are most easily detected on lymphocytes. Essential to immunity, these antigens determine the degree of histocompatibility between transplant recipients and donors. Generally, HLA testing benefits patients receiving massive or multiple long-term transfusions, or frequent transfusions during a limited illness. Such patients may develop antibodies to the donor platelets and WBCs present in all donor RBC products. Most of these antigen-antibody reactions involve the histocompatibility system.

Also expect to seek an HLA evaluation for patients scheduled to receive platelet and WBC transfusions, for those with severe or refractory febrile transfusion reactions, and for those undergoing organ transplantation. The HLA system is responsible for graft rejection and may be associated with host defense against cancer. It may also be involved when WBCs or platelets fail to multiply after being transfused. If this happens, the HLA system could trigger a fatal immune reaction in the patient.

Administering transfusion

After the blood or blood product has been tested and typed, your primary responsibility is to prevent a potentially fatal hemolytic reaction by making sure the patient receives the correct blood or blood product. Before administering any blood or blood product, double-check the patient's name, medical record number, ABO and Rh status (and other compatibility factors), and blood bank identification number against the label on the blood bag. Also check the expiration date on the bag.

Ask another nurse or doctor to

verify all information, according to hospital policy. (Some hospitals routinely require double identification.) Make sure both you and the nurse or doctor who checked the blood or blood product sign the blood confirmation slip. If even a slight discrepancy exists, *do not* administer the blood or blood product. Instead, immediately notify the blood bank.

Next, inspect the blood or blood product to detect any abnormalities. Then confirm the patient's identity by checking the name, room number, and bed number on his wristband. After that, teach your patient about the transfusion and its therapeutic benefits. (See *Transfusion teaching topics.*) If appropriate, you may discuss voluntary blood donations with the patient and his family.

You'll follow the same basic procedure whether you transfuse whole blood, cellular components, plasma, or plasma fractions. Your selection of equipment, however, will depend on the product being transfused. So will some of the specific precautions you take and the care measures you perform.

Beside knowing how to perform standard transfusion procedures, you may also need to know how to use other methods of therapy, such as hemapheresis and autotransfusion. You must also be prepared to meet the special needs of pediatric, elderly, and home care patients who require transfusion.

Transfusing whole blood and cellular components

Before a transfusion, you need to send for the blood or cellular components, as ordered, and gather and set up the appropriate equipment. (If your patient is receiving whole blood or packed RBCs, don't send for

CHECKLIST

Transfusion teaching topics

When teaching your patient what to expect before, during, and after the transfusion, be sure to cover these topics:
☐ Explain the need for the transfusion, describing the inadequacy of non-human derivatives such as dextran (if appropriate), and the potential consequences of not having the transfusion.
☐ Describe the components the patient will receive and the benefits.
☐ Explain the possible adverse reactions of the transfusion.
☐ Discuss the patient's anticipated response to the transfusion and the potential for future transfusions.
☐ Detail the specific steps of the transfusion.
☐ Explain to the patient what he should do during the procedure.

the blood until just before you gather the equipment; RBCs deteriorate after 2 hours at room temperature.)

Selecting blood or cellular components. The patient's condition determines the type of transfusion he needs. (See *Guide to blood components,* pages 160 to 162.) To replenish decreased blood volume or to boost the blood's oxygen-carrying capacity, you'll probably transfuse either whole blood or packed RBCs. Both choices treat decreased hemoglobin level and hematocrit, but massive blood loss—for example, from trauma or vascular or cardiac surgery—generally requires whole blood transfusion.

Washed cells, such as leukocyte-poor RBCs, are similar to packed RBCs in that 80% of the plasma has

(Text continues on page 162.)

Guide to blood components

BLOOD COMPONENT	INDICATIONS	NURSING CONSIDERATIONS
Whole blood Complete (pure) blood *Volume:* 500 ml	• To restore blood volume in hemorrhaging, trauma, or burn patients	• Cross-typing: ABO identical. Group A receives A; group B receives B; group AB receives AB; group O receives O. Rh match. • Use straight-line or Y-type I.V. set; infuse over 2 to 4 hours. • Whole blood is seldom administered because its components can be extracted and administered separately. • Contraindicated when patient doesn't or can't tolerate the circulatory volume.
Packed red blood cells (RBCs) Same RBC mass as whole blood with 80% of the plasma removed *Volume:* 250 ml	• To restore or maintain oxygen-carrying capacity • To correct anemia and surgical blood loss • To increase RBC mass	• Cross-typing: Group A receives A or O; group B receives B or O; group AB receives AB, A, B, O; group O receives O. Rh match. • Use straight-line or Y-type I.V. set; infuse over 1½ to 4 hours. • RBCs have the same oxygen-carrying capacity as whole blood without the hazards of volume overload. • Using packed RBCs avoids potassium and ammonia buildup that sometimes occurs in the plasma of stored blood. • Packed RBCs shouldn't be used for anemic conditions correctable by nutrition or drug therapy.
Leukocyte-poor RBCs Same as packed RBCs except leukocytes (70%) are removed *Volume:* 200 ml	• Same as packed RBCs • To prevent febrile reactions from leukocyte antibodies • To treat immunosuppressed patients	• Cross-typing: Same as packed RBCs. Rh match. • Use straight-line or Y-type I.V. set. May require a Pall filter (40 micron filter) for hard-spun, leukocyte-poor RBCs. Infuse over 1½ to 4 hours. • Other considerations same as for packed RBCs.
White blood cells (leukocytes) Whole blood with all the RBCs and 80% of the supernatant plasma removed *Volume:* 150 ml	• To treat a patient with life-threatening granulocytopenia (granulocyte count usually less than 500/mm³) who's not responding to antibiotics (especially if he has positive blood cultures or persistent fever greater than 101° F [38.3° C])	• Cross-typing: Same as packed RBCs. Rh match. Preferably human leukocyte antigen (HLA) compatible but not necessary unless patient is HLA sensitized from previous transfusions. • Use straight-line set with standard in-line blood filter. Dosage is 1 unit daily for 5 days or until infection clears. • WBC infusion induces fever and chills. Administer an antipyretic if fever occurs, but don't discontinue transfusion. Flow rate may be reduced for patient comfort. • Give transfusion in conjunction with antibiotics to treat infection.

Guide to blood components (continued)

BLOOD COMPONENT	INDICATIONS	NURSING CONSIDERATIONS
Platelets Platelet sediment from RBCs or plasma *Volume:* 35 to 50 ml/unit; 1 unit of platelets = 7 × 10⁷ platelets	• To treat thrombocytopenia caused by decreased platelet production, increased platelet destruction, or massive transfusion of stored blood • To treat acute leukemia and marrow aplasia • To restore platelet count in a preoperative patient with a count of 100,000/mm³ or less	• Cross-typing: ABO compatibility not necessary but preferable with repeated platelet transfusions. Rh match preferred. • Use a component drip administration set; infuse 100 ml over 15 minutes. • Patients with a history of platelet reaction require premedication with antipyretics and antihistamines. • Avoid administering platelets when the patient has a fever. • A blood platelet count may be ordered 1 hour after platelet transfusion to determine platelet transfusion increments. • Platelet transfusions usually aren't indicated for conditions of accelerated platelet destruction, such as idiopathic thrombocytopenia purpura, or drug-induced thrombocytopenia.
Fresh frozen plasma (FFP) Uncoagulated plasma separated from RBCs. FFP is rich in coagulation factors V, VIII, IX. *Volume:* 200 to 250 ml	• To expand plasma volume • To treat postsurgical hemorrhage or shock • To correct an undetermined coagulation factor deficiency • To replace a specific factor when that factor alone isn't available • To correct factor deficiencies resulting from hepatic disease	• Cross-typing: Same as for platelets. • Use straight-line set and administer rapidly. • Large-volume transfusions of FFP may require correction for hypocalcemia. Citric acid in FFP binds calcium.
Albumin 5% (buffered saline); albumin 25% (salt-poor) Human albumin is a small plasma protein prepared by fractionation of pooled plasma. *Volume:* 5% = 12.5 g/250 ml; 25% = 12.5 g/50 ml	• To replace volume in treatment of shock from burns, trauma, surgery, or infections • To replace volume and prevent marked hemoconcentration • To treat hypoproteinemia (with or without edema)	• Cross-typing: Unnecessary. • Use a straight-line set at a rate and volume dependent on the patient's condition and response. • Reactions to albumin (fever, chills, nausea) are rare. • Shouldn't be mixed with protein hydrolysates and alcohol solutions. • Often given as a volume expander until cross matching for whole blood is complete. • Contraindicated in severe anemia and administered cautiously in cardiac and pulmonary disease because of risk of congestive heart failure from circulatory overload.

(continued)

Guide to blood components *(continued)*

BLOOD COMPONENT	INDICATIONS	NURSING CONSIDERATIONS
Factor VIII (cryo-precipitate) Cold insoluble portion of plasma recovered from FFP. *Volume:* approximately 30 ml (freeze dried)	• To treat a patient with hemophilia A • To control bleeding associated with Factor VIII deficiency • To replace fibrinogen or Factor VIII	• Cross-typing: ABO compatibility not necessary but preferable. • Use the manufacturer-supplied administration set; administer with a filter. Standard dose recommended for treatment of acute bleeding episodes in hemophilia is 15 to 20 units/kg. • Half-life of Factor VIII (8 to 10 hours) necessitates repeat transfusions at these intervals to maintain normal levels.
Factors II, VII, IX, X complex (prothrombin complex) Lyophilized commercially-prepared solution drawn from pooled plasma	• To treat a congenital Factor V deficiency and other bleeding disorders resulting from an acquired deficiency of Factors II, VII, IX, and X	• Cross-typing: No ABO/Rh matching. • Use a straight-line set; dosage based on desired level and patient's body weight. • Very high risk of hepatitis. • Coagulation assays are performed before administration and at suitable intervals during treatment. • Contraindicated when the patient has hepatic disease resulting in fibrinolysis. • Contraindicated when the patient has intravascular coagulation and isn't undergoing heparin therapy.

been removed. Unlike packed RBCs, however, they've also been rinsed with a special solution that removes WBCs and platelets. Washed cells replenish the blood's oxygen-carrying capacity in patients who have been previously sensitized by transfusions.

You may be ordered to transfuse WBCs, primarily granulocytes, to treat septicemia and other life-threatening infections that don't respond to routine therapies—especially if these complications occur in severely granulocytopenic patients. Because some RBCs normally exist in WBC concentrates, the blood is tested for compatibility (ABO, Rh type, and HLA when possible). To ensure the effectiveness of therapy, repeat the daily administration of WBCs for 4 to 5 days or longer, as ordered.

Selecting the equipment. Gather the following equipment: a straight-line blood administration set (filter and tubing with drip chamber for blood), a three-way stopcock, a regular I.V. administration set, and clamps. Or you can use a Y-type blood administration set. You'll also need 250 ml of saline solution, an I.V. pole, clean gloves, a gown, a mask, and either whole blood, packed RBCs, washed RBCs, or WBC concentrates, as ordered. You may also need venipuncture equipment.

Some doctors use lactated Ringer's solution instead of saline solution as a diluent for transfusions. Others don't use lactated Ringer's because the calcium chloride in the solution may cause clotting. Generally, expect to use lactated Ringer's solution only in certain controlled areas, such as an operating room or a trauma center.

• *Filters.* Use blood filters on all blood products to avoid infusing any fibrin clots that have formed in the blood bag. Filters come in many types, each with unique features and indications. The standard blood administration set comes with a 170-micron filter, which removes agglutinates of platelets, leukocytes, and large fibrin strands. This filter doesn't remove smaller particles, called microaggregates, which are thought to form after only a few days of blood storage and can contribute to microemboli in the lungs. To remove microaggregates, the doctor may order a 20- or 40-micron filter.

Although a microaggregate filter removes smaller particles, it also costs more, may cause clots, and may slow the infusion rate—a particular problem during massive, rapid transfusion. If you use a microaggregate filter, remember to replace it after administering 2 units of blood, or if more than 1 hour elapses between transfusions. *Never* use a microaggregate filter to transfuse WBC concentrates or platelets; the filter will trap them.

• *Blood warmer.* Besides the standard transfusion equipment, the doctor may also order a blood warmer. Expect to use a blood warmer to prevent or treat hypothermia—for example, from a massive transfusion or immediately after surgery. Also use a blood warmer when special antibodies, called cold agglutinins, are present and could cause RBC aggregation if infused cold. In many hospitals, a blood warmer is also used to prevent arrhythmias when giving a transfusion through a CV line. (See *Using a dry-heat blood warmer,* page 164.)

• *Infusion pump.* In most hospitals,

an infusion pump is used to regulate the administration of blood and blood products. Always check the manufacturer's instructions to determine if the specific pump can be used to administer blood or blood products.

Starting the transfusion. First, wash your hands and put on the gloves, gown, and mask. If you're using a straight-line set, insert the set's tubing spike into the bag of saline solution. Hang the bag on the I.V. pole, and prime the filter and tubing with saline solution to reduce the risk of microclots forming in the tubing. Leave the bag of saline solution attached to the tubing until you're ready to start the transfusion.

As discussed earlier, you must check the expiration date of the blood or cellular component. Also, double-check that you're giving the right blood or cellular component to the right patient. Observe the blood or cellular component for abnormal color, RBC clumping, gas bubbles, and extraneous material.

When you're ready to start the transfusion, you'll need to prepare the equipment. If you're using a *straight-line set*, disconnect the blood administration set from the saline solution and clamp the open port of the saline solution. Then open the port on the blood bag and insert the spike on the blood administration set into the port. Next, remove the clamp from the saline solution and insert the spike on the regular administration set into the bag of saline solution and prime the line. After that, turn the three-way stopcock to the off position and connect it to the end of the blood tubing. Then connect the saline solution to the stopcock.

If you're using a *Y-type set*, close

Using a dry-heat blood warmer

A rapid transfusion of cold blood can lead to hypothermia and may cause arrhythmias. So, depending on your hospital's policy, you may use a dry-heat blood warmer for massive, rapid transfusions and for exchange transfusions in neonates. You can also use this device for transfusions in patients with increased cold agglutinin titers. The warmer maintains a constant temperature of 98.6° F (37° C). To use it:

• Plug in the device and prepare the patient and equipment. After eliminating the air from the administration set, close the main flow clamp.

• Insert the warming bag into the blood warmer. Match the bottom lead (for the blood line) and the top lead (for the patient) to the corresponding openings in the blood warmer. (The top lead connector is shown here; the bottom lead connector, which is on the back of device, isn't shown.) Note that the top lead has a special outlet chamber attached to it. Mount the warming bag on the support pins, keeping the bag flat against the back panel. Secure the pins.

• Close the blood warmer door and secure the latch. Turn the machine on, and allow it to operate for at least 2 minutes to warm the blood to 98.6° F. Avoid opening the door until the transfusion is completed. Otherwise, you'll break the vacuum, then you must replace the warming bag.

• While the blood warms, connect the blood line adapter to the female adapter on the bottom lead. After the desired temperature is achieved, open the saline line clamp and the main flow clamp to fill the bag with normal saline solution. Squeeze the outlet chamber until it's flat; continue to hold the chamber. When saline solution appears in the chamber, close the main flow clamp and release the chamber. The chamber then automatically fills

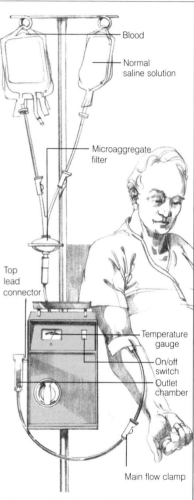

halfway with saline solution.

• Remove the adapter cover on the top lead and open the clamp. Expel residual air from the line. Then, close the clamp and recap the line. Proceed as you would when administering blood with a Y-type set.

all the clamps on the set. Then insert the spike of the line you're using for the saline solution into the bag of saline solution. Next, open the port on the blood bag and insert the spike of the line you're using to administer the blood or cellular component into the port. Hang the saline solution and blood or cellular component on the I.V. pole, open the clamp on the line of saline solution, and squeeze the drip chamber until it's half full of saline solution. Then remove the adapter cover at the tip of the blood administration set, open the main flow clamp, and prime the tubing with saline solution. Close the clamp and recap the adapter.

To transfuse the blood or cellular component, follow these steps:

• Explain the procedure to the patient.

• Take the patient's vital signs to serve as baseline values. Recheck vital signs after 15 minutes (or according to hospital policy).

• If the patient doesn't have an I.V. line in place, perform a venipuncture, preferably using either an 18G catheter or a 19G needle. Avoid using an existing line with a needle or catheter lumen that's smaller than 20G.

• Attach the prepared blood administration set to the venipuncture device and flush it with saline solution. If you're using a straight-line set with a stopcock, you'll turn the stopcock so the saline solution can run through and flush the device. If you're using a Y-type set, you'll open both the clamp on the saline solution line and the main flow clamp.

• If you're administering whole blood or WBCs, gently invert the bag several times to mix the cells. (During the transfusion, gently agitate the bag to prevent settle-ment of the viscous cells.)

• After you've flushed the venipuncture device, turn the stopcock to close the saline solution line and open the blood line if you're using a straight-line set. Or close the clamp to stop the saline solution and open the clamp between the blood bag and the patient if you're using a Y-type set.

• Then adjust the flow clamp closest to the patient to deliver a slow rate (usually about 20 gtt/minute) for the first 10 to 30 minutes. The type of blood product given and the patient's clinical condition determine the rate of transfusion. A unit of RBCs may be given over a period of between 1 and 4 hours; platelets and coagulation factors may be given more quickly than RBCs or granulocytes. Usually, you won't take any longer than 4 hours because the risk of contamination and sepsis increases after that. Discard or return to the blood bank any blood or blood products not given within this time, as hospital policy directs.

• Assess the patient and monitor vital signs according to hospital policy. If you detect signs of a transfusion reaction, such as fever, chills, or nausea, quickly check and record the patient's vital signs. Then, stop the transfusion, start infusing the saline solution at a keep-vein-open rate, and notify the doctor.

• If no signs of a reaction appear within 30 minutes, adjust the flow clamp to achieve the ordered infusion rate. Or you can open the clamp completely and adjust the infusion rate by raising or lowering the blood bag. This method reduces the risk of hemolysis from pressure on the tubing.

• Check the infusion rate frequently; it often slows after the initial infu-

Transfusing blood under pressure

Rapid blood replacement requires transfusing blood under pressure. First, select the proper equipment—a pressure cuff or a positive-pressure set. The pressure cuff is placed over the blood bag like a sleeve and inflated, as shown. The pressure gauge, attached to the cuff, is calibrated in millimeters of mercury. The positive-pressure set is a gravity administration set containing a built-in pressure chamber that increases the flow rate when the chamber is compressed, as shown.

To use either of these devices, prepare the patient and set up the equipment as you would with a straight-line blood administration set. Prime the filter and tubing with saline solution to remove all air from the administration set. Connect the tubing to the needle or catheter hub. During the transfusion, watch the patient closely for complications, such as extravasation, which can occur rapidly.

Pressure cuff
To use this device:
• Insert your hand into the pressure cuff sleeve and pull the blood bag up through the center opening. Then, grasp one loop of the sleeve, slip it through the blood bag loop, and pull

PRESSURE CUFF

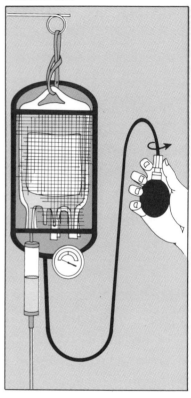

sion of saline solution.
• If you use a pressure bag to encase the blood or blood product and increase the rate of infusion, be aware that excessive pressure may develop, leading to broken blood vessels and extravasation, with hematoma and hemolysis of the infusing RBCs. (See *Transfusing blood under pressure.*)
• After the transfusion, flush the blood line with 5 to 10 ml of saline solution. On a straight-line set, turn the stopcock to close the blood line and open the saline solution line. On a Y-type set, close the clamp on the blood line and open the clamp on the saline line. Then either reconnect the original I.V. fluid or remove the I.V. line.
• Return the empty blood bag to the blood bank, according to hospital policy. Be sure to discard the tubing and filter.

POSITIVE-PRESSURE SET

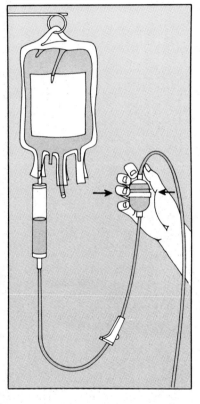

the other sleeve loop through it.
• Hang the blood bag on the I.V. pole. Open the flow clamp on the tubing (not shown).
• To set the flow rate, turn the screw clamp on the pressure cuff counterclockwise. Compress the pressure bulb of the cuff to inflate the bag until you achieve the desired flow rate. Then, turn the screw clamp clockwise to maintain this constant flow rate.
• As the blood bag empties, the pressure decreases, so check the flow rate regularly and adjust the pressure in the pressure cuff as necessary to maintain a consistent flow rate. But don't allow the cuff needle to exceed 300 mm Hg. Excessively high pressure may cause hemolysis.

Positive-pressure set
To use this device:
• Open the upper and lower flow clamps on the administration set.
• Manually compress and release the pump chamber to force blood down the tubing and to the patient. Allow the pump chamber to refill completely before compressing it again.
• Continue to compress and release the chamber until the blood bag empties or until rapid administration is no longer necessary.

• Reassess the patient's condition and take his vital signs.
• Record the date and time of the transfusion, the type and amount of blood transfused, the patient's vital signs, and your efforts to check all the identifying data. Also document any transfusion reaction and treatment.
Note: Don't administer drugs during the transfusion; otherwise, you may not be able to identify the

source of an adverse reaction.

Transfusing plasma and plasma fractions
Transfusion of plasma and its fractions can correct blood deficiencies, such as low platelet count; prevent disease, such as hepatitis; and control bleeding tendencies. Before transfusion, obtain the plasma or plasma fractions, as ordered, and select and set up the equipment.

Selecting the plasma or plasma fractions. Transfusion of platelets suspended in 30 to 50 ml of plasma can correct an extremely low platelet count (below 20,000 to 50,000/mm³), as may occur in patients with hematologic disease, such as aplastic anemia and leukemia, and in those receiving antineoplastic chemotherapy. The prevention or control of bleeding will often require a large quantity of platelets — typically 4 or more units in an adult.

Plasma substitutes lack oxygen-carrying and hemostatic properties, but you can use them to maintain circulatory volume in an emergency, such as acute hemorrhage and shock. This gives you time to get the patient's blood typed and cross matched or the injury repaired. Depending on the circumstances, you may give a synthetic volume expander, such as dextran in saline solution, or a natural volume expander, such as plasma protein fraction and albumin.

Gamma globulin, the antibody-containing portion of plasma obtained by chemical fractionation of pooled plasma, may be used to prevent infectious hepatitis (type A), rubella, mumps, pertussis, and tetanus (if given before clinical symptoms develop). Gamma globulin may also be used to treat hypogammaglobulinemia and agammaglobulinemia. It's used experimentally to treat idiopathic thrombocytopenia purpura. Gamma globulin should not be given to patients with known hypersensitivity to it or to an anti-immunoglobulin (anti-IgA) antibody. Other plasma fractions include cryoprecipitate and prothrombin complex.

Selecting the equipment. Gather the following equipment: a straight-line blood administration set, a three-way stopcock, a regular I.V. administration set, and a clamp. Or you could use a Y-type blood administration set. No matter which administration set you use, it should have a 170-micron or larger filter. If you're administering platelets or cryoprecipitate, use a component drip administration set instead of the Y-type or straight-line set.

You'll also need saline solution, an I.V. pole, clean gloves, a gown, a mask, and the plasma or plasma fractions, as ordered. You may need venipuncture equipment.

Note: Never use a microaggregate filter to infuse platelets or plasma; the filter may remove essential components from the transfusion.

Starting the transfusion. First, wash your hands and put on the clean gloves, gown, and mask. Then prepare the equipment as described above, unless you're using a component drip administration set for platelets or cryoprecipitate. For these components, you won't prime with saline solution. That's because the saline could destroy the platelets or cryoprecipitate. Instead, you'll insert the spike of the component drip administration set into the component bag, hang the bag on the I.V. pole, and carefully prime the set with the platelets or cryoprecipitate.

As discussed earlier, you must check the expiration date of the plasma or plasma fraction. Also, double-check that you're giving the right plasma or plasma fraction to the right patient. Then inspect the plasma or plasma fraction for cloudiness and turbidity, and look for leaks in the plastic bag.

Be sure to use fresh frozen plasma (FFP) within 4 hours because it does not contain preservatives. When transfusing a Factor VIII or prothrombin preparation, carefully reconstitute it according to the manufacturer's directions, if the pharmacy hasn't already prepared it.

To transfuse the plasma or plasma fraction, follow these steps:
• Explain the procedure to the patient.
• Obtain baseline vital signs and continue to check vital signs frequently, according to hospital policy.
• If the patient doesn't have an I.V. line in place, perform a venipuncture, preferably using an 18G catheter or a 19G needle. Avoid using an existing line if the needle or catheter lumen is smaller than 20G.
• Attach the plasma, FFP, albumin, Factor VIII concentrate, prothrombin complex, platelets, or cryoprecipitate to the patient's venipuncture device and flush it with saline solution, as described above — unless you're administering platelets or cryoprecipitate. In that case, flush the device with 5 ml of saline solution *before* attaching the component administration set.
• Begin the transfusion and adjust the flow rate as ordered.
• Take the patient's vital signs and assess him frequently for signs of a transfusion reaction, such as fever, chills, or nausea. Transfusion reactions occur more commonly with the administration of platelets, WBCs, and cryoprecipitate than with whole blood, RBCs, or plasma. If a reaction occurs, quickly check and record the patient's vital signs. Then, stop the transfusion, start the infusion of saline solution at a keep-vein-open rate, and notify the doctor.
• After the infusion, flush the line with 20 to 30 ml of saline solution. Then disconnect the I.V. line. If therapy will continue, hang the original I.V. solution and adjust the flow rate, as ordered.

• Record the type and amount of plasma or plasma fraction administered, duration of transfusion, baseline vital signs, and any adverse reactions.
• *Using a component syringe set.* As an alternative to the component drip set, you can use a component syringe set to give platelets or cryoprecipitate. To do so, follow these steps:
• Close both clamps on the syringe set. Then, open the port of the platelet or cryoprecipitate bag by pulling back the tabs. Next, remove the protective cover of the administration set spike. Always use the administration set supplied by the manufacturer; it contains a small concealed filter that removes particles and other contaminants.
• Using a twisting motion, insert the administration set spike into the port. Then, attach the syringe to the luer-tip port of the syringe administration set.
• Attach a three-way stopcock to the patient end of the syringe administration set.
• Open the clamp above the Y-connector and draw up to 50 ml of platelets or cryoprecipitate into the syringe. Close the clamp and then open it below the Y-connector. Holding the syringe upright, prime the tubing with the platelets or cryoprecipitate, and close the clamp.
• Connect the line to the patient's venipuncture device and infuse the platelets or cryoprecipitate at the ordered rate.
• Check frequently for signs of bleeding, and instruct the patient to report even slight bleeding.
• After the infusion, flush the line with 20 to 30 ml of saline solution. Next, disconnect the I.V. line or, if therapy will continue, hang the original I.V. solution and adjust the flow rate, as ordered.

• Record the amount of platelets or cryoprecipitate given, the duration of the transfusion, baseline vital signs, and any adverse reactions.

Special considerations. If albumin has been diluted or added to another solution, use it as soon as possible to prevent bacterial growth. If you have difficulty establishing the flow of an albumin infusion, suspect an air lock in the vent on the tubing spike. Correct this by wiping the container's rubber stopper with an alcohol swab and inserting a 20G 1″ needle. If this doesn't work, change the tubing. If you still can't establish the flow, get a new container of albumin and a new administration set, and return the old one.

If the patient requires whole blood or packed RBCs after the plasma transfusion, you can still administer the plasma with either a straight-line or Y-type set. After you've given the plasma, maintain the I.V. line with saline solution at a keep-vein-open rate until you're ready to transfuse the blood.

Administer any additional bags of platelets by removing the component drip administration set spike and inserting it in the new bag. Close the clamp and attach the new bag before the drip chamber empties to keep air from entering the line. Because platelet transfusion requires frequent bag changes and manipulation of the line, schedule your daily patient care duties around these steps.

Specialized transfusions

Hemapheresis and autotransfusion are two specialized means of administering blood. Hemapheresis involves collecting and removing specific blood components, and then returning the remaining blood constituents to the donor. Autotransfu-

sion involves collecting, filtering, and reinfusing the patient's own blood. The doctor will order autotransfusion after a traumatic injury and before, during, and after surgery.

Both hemapheresis and autotransfusion must be performed by skilled personnel. Nurses who are familiar with the procedures may monitor and evaluate a patient's condition throughout the transfusion.

Precautions and complications

If you're caring for a pediatric or elderly patient who needs a transfusion, you must be aware of certain precautions. The same holds true if you're caring for a patient who'll be receiving a transfusion at home. What's more, during a transfusion for *any* patient, you must check scrupulously for potential complications, such as transfusion reaction.

Patients with special needs

Pediatric, elderly, and home care patients all require special care during therapy. For instance, transfusing blood into neonates requires highly specialized training because their physiologic requirements differ vastly from those of the older infant, child, or adult.

Pediatric patients. Transfusions in children differ significantly from transfusions in adults. Blood units for pediatric patients are prepared in half-unit packs, and you'll probably use a 24G or 22G thin-walled catheter or a 23G or 21G butterfly needle to administer the blood. The rate of the infusion also differs.

Usually, a child receives 5% to 10% of the total transfusion in the first 15 minutes of therapy. To maintain the correct flow rate, be sure to use an infusion pump.

Closely monitor the child throughout the transfusion, particularly during the first 15 minutes to detect early signs of a reaction. Use a blood warmer during the transfusion to prevent hypothermia and cardiac arrhythmias, especially if you're administering blood through a CV line.

A child's normal circulating blood volume determines the amount of blood transfused. The average blood volume for children and infants older than 1 month is 75 ml/kg. The proportion of blood volume to body weight decreases with age.

In massive hemorrhage and shock, the indications for blood component transfusion remain similar to those for adults, although accurate assessment of blood loss is more difficult. Draw blood from a central vein to get a more accurate hemoglobin level and hematocrit, or use blood pressure readings to determine blood volume. (See *Detecting pediatric volume depletion.*)

Whenever you transfuse blood in an infant or child, explain the procedure, its purpose, and the possible complications to the parents; if appropriate, also include the child in the explanation. Ask the parents for the child's transfusion history and obtain their consent.

Elderly patients. An elderly patient with preexisting heart disease may be unable to tolerate rapid transfusion of an entire unit of blood without exhibiting signs of congestive heart failure, such as shortness of breath. Such a patient may be better able to tolerate half-unit blood transfusions.

Detecting pediatric volume depletion

Normal systolic blood pressure varies with a child's age. This chart shows the corresponding ages and systolic readings that indicate a child has lost more than 30% of his blood volume.

AGE RANGE	SYSTOLIC BLOOD PRESSURE
Under age 4	< 65 mm Hg
Ages 5 to 8	< 75 mm Hg
Ages 9 to 12	< 85 mm Hg
Adolescent	< 95 mm Hg

Age-related slowing of the immune system places the older adult patient at risk for delayed inflammatory transfusion reactions. This can result in a more severe reaction because greater quantities of blood products transfuse before signs or symptoms appear. Also, an elderly patient tends to be less resistant to infection.

Home care patients. Standards established by the American Association of Blood Banks, in accordance with federal, state, and local regulations, allow a doctor to order transfusions of blood products (not whole blood) for home care patients. To qualify, a patient must be unable to leave his home without assistance and must have received previous transfusions without difficulties.

Complications

Administering a transfusion involves taking steps to prevent complications—and knowing how to manage them when they arise. Transfusion-related complications can be imme-

Correcting transfusion problems

A patient who receives excellent care can still encounter problems during a transfusion. Here's how to proceed when common transfusion problems occur.

If the transfusion stops:
• Check that the I.V. container is at least 3 feet (1 m) above the level of the I.V. site.
• Make sure the flow clamp is open.
• Make sure the blood completely covers the filter. If it doesn't, squeeze the drip chamber until it does, as shown below.

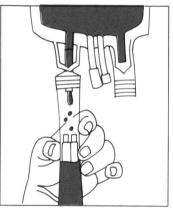

• Gently rock the bag back and forth, agitating any blood cells that may have settled on the bottom.
• Untape the dressing over the I.V. site to check the placement of the needle in the vein. Reposition the needle, if necessary.
• If using a straight-line blood administration set, flush the line with saline solution and restart the transfusion. If

using a Y-type blood administration set, close the flow clamp to the patient and lower the blood bag. Next, open the saline clamp and allow some saline solution to flow into the blood bag. Rehang the blood bag, open the flow clamp to the patient, and reset the flow rate.

If a hematoma develops at the I.V. site:
• Immediately stop the infusion.
• Remove the needle or catheter and cap the tubing with a new needle and guard.
• Notify the doctor and expect to place ice on the site for 24 hours; after that, you'll apply warm compresses.
• Promote reabsorption of the hematoma by having the patient gently exercise the affected limb.
• Document your observations and actions.

If the blood bag empties before the next one arrives:
• Hang a container of saline solution and administer it slowly.
• If using a Y-type set, close the blood line clamp, open the saline clamp, and let the saline solution run slowly until the new blood arrives. Make sure you decrease the flow rate or clamp the line before attaching the new unit of blood.

diate, as with a transfusion reaction, or delayed, as with a transmittable infectious disease. They can also stem from mechanical malfunction or other problems with the transfusion equipment. (See *Correcting*

transfusion problems.)
    Certain complications, such as hypothermia, bleeding tendencies, and hemosiderosis, typically result from multiple or massive transfu-

(*Text continues on page 176.*)

COMPLICATIONS

 Managing transfusion reactions

Transfusion of processed blood products puts a patient at risk for certain complications, such as hemosiderosis and hypothermia. The first part of this chart tells
you how to recognize the five types of transfusion reactions and how to intervene
after you stop the infusion. The second part of this chart tells you how to recognize, treat, and prevent some common complications of multiple transfusions.

REACTION	SIGNS AND SYMPTOMS	NURSING INTERVENTIONS
Reactions from any transfusion		
Hemolytic *Causes:* ● ABO or Rh incompati- bility ● Intra-donor incompati- bility ● Improper storage of blood	● Shaking, chills, fever, nausea, vomiting, chest pain, dyspnea, hypoten- sion, oliguria, hemoglo- binuria, flank pain, abnormal bleeding ● May progress to shock and renal failure	● Monitor blood pressure. ● Treat shock as indicated by pa- tient's condition, using I.V. fluids, ox- ygen, epinephrine, a diuretic, and a vasopressor. ● Obtain posttransfusion reaction blood and urine samples for evalua- tion. ● Observe for signs of hemorrhage resulting from disseminated intra- vascular coagulation. *Prevention:* ● Before transfusion, check donor and recipient blood types to ensure blood compatibility; also identify pa- tient with another nurse or doctor present. ● Transfuse blood slowly for first 15 to 20 minutes; closely observe pa- tient for the first 20 minutes of the transfusion.
Febrile *Cause:* ● Presence of bacterial lipopolysaccharides	● Fever, chills, head- ache, flank pain	● Relieve symptoms with an antipy- retic, antihistamine, or meperidine (Demerol). *Prevention:* ● Premedicate with an antipyretic, antihistamine, and possibly a ste- roid. ● Use leukocyte-poor or washed red blood cells (RBCs).
Allergic *Cause:* ● Allergen in donor's blood	● Pruritus, urticaria, fe- ver, chills, nausea, vom- iting, facial swelling, wheezing, laryngeal edema ● May progress to ana- phylactic reaction	● Administer antihistamines. ● Monitor for anaphylactic reaction and administer epinephrine and ste- roids, if indicated. *Prevention:* ● Premedicate with antihistamine if patient has a history of allergic re- actions. ● Observe patient closely for the first 20 minutes of the transfusion.

(continued)

COMPLICATIONS

Managing transfusion reactions *(continued)*

REACTION	SIGNS AND SYMPTOMS	NURSING INTERVENTIONS
Plasma protein incompatibility *Cause:* • IgA incompatibility	• Flushing, abdominal pain, diarrhea, chills, fever, dyspnea, hypotension	• Treat for shock by administering oxygen, fluids, epinephrine, and possibly a steroid, as ordered. *Prevention:* • Transfuse only IgA-deficient blood or well-washed RBCs.
Bacterial contamination *Cause:* • Presence of gram-negative organisms that can survive cold species of *Pseudomonas*	• Chills, fever, vomiting, abdominal cramping, diarrhea, shock, signs of renal failure	• Treat with broad-spectrum antibiotic and steroid. *Prevention:* • Observe blood before transfusion for gas, clots, and dark purple color. • Use air-free, touch-free method to draw and deliver blood. • Maintain strict storage control. • Change blood tubing and filter every 4 hours. • Infuse each unit of blood over 2 to 4 hours; terminate the infusion if the time period exceeds 4 hours. • Maintain sterile technique when administering blood products.

Reactions from multiple transfusions

Hemosiderosis *Cause:* • Increased hemosiderin (iron-containing pigment) from RBC destruction, especially after receiving chronic transfusions	• Iron plasma level greater than 200 mg/dl	• Perform a phlebotomy to remove excess iron. *Prevention:* • Administer blood only when absolutely necessary.
Bleeding tendencies *Cause:* • Low platelet count in stored blood, causing dilutional thrombocytopenia	• Abnormal bleeding and oozing from cut or break in skin surface	• Administer platelets. • Monitor platelet count. *Prevention:* • Use only fresh blood (less than 7 days old) when possible.
Elevated blood ammonia level *Cause:* • Increased level of ammonia in stored blood	• Forgetfulness, confusion	• Monitor ammonia level. • Decrease the amount of protein in the diet. • If indicated, give neomycin sulfate. *Prevention:* • Use only RBCs, fresh frozen plasma, or fresh blood, especially if patient has hepatic disease.

Managing transfusion reactions *(continued)*

REACTION	SIGNS AND SYMPTOMS	NURSING INTERVENTIONS
Increased oxygen affinity for hemoglobin *Cause:* • Decreased level of 2,3 DPG in stored blood, causing an increase in the oxygen's hemoglobin affinity. When this occurs, oxygen stays in the patient's bloodstream and isn't released into his tissues.	• Depressed respiratory rate, especially in patients with chronic lung disease	• Monitor arterial blood gas (ABG) levels and give respiratory support as needed. *Prevention:* • Use only RBCs or fresh blood if possible.
Hypothermia *Cause:* • Rapid infusion of large amounts of cold blood, which decreases myocardial temperature	• Shaking chills, hypotension, ventricular fibrillation • Cardiac arrest, if core temperature falls below 86° F (30° C)	• Stop transfusion. • Warm patient with blankets. • Obtain an electrocardiogram (ECG). *Prevention:* • Warm blood to 95° to 98.6° F (35° to 37° C), especially before massive transfusions.
Hypocalcemia *Cause:* • Citrate toxicity occurs when citrate-treated blood is infused rapidly. Citrate binds with calcium, causing a calcium deficiency, or normal citrate metabolism becomes hindered by hepatic disease.	• Tingling in fingers, muscle cramps, nausea, vomiting, hypotension, cardiac arrhythmias, convulsions	• Slow or stop transfusion, depending on reaction. Expect a worse reaction in hypothermic patients or patients with elevated potassium levels. • Slowly administer calcium gluconate I.V. *Prevention:* • Infuse blood slowly. • Monitor potassium and calcium levels. • Use blood less than 2 days old if administering multiple units.
Potassium intoxication *Cause:* • An abnormally high level of potassium in stored plasma caused by RBC lysis	• Intestinal colic, diarrhea, muscle twitching, oliguria, renal failure, ECG changes with tall peaked T waves, bradycardia proceeding to cardiac standstill	• Obtain an ECG. • Administer sodium polystyrene sulfonate (Kayexalate) orally or by enema. *Prevention:* • Use fresh blood when administering massive transfusions.

sions. (See *Managing transfusion reactions,* pages 173 to 175.) Transfusions of blood products, which have been processed and preserved, put the patient at risk, especially when he receives frequent transfusions of large amounts.

Transfusion reactions. Usually attributed to major antigen-antibody reactions, transfusion reactions occur within 96 hours after the transfusion begins. Whenever you detect signs or symptoms of a transfusion reaction, immediately stop the transfusion. Then proceed as follows:
• Change the I.V. tubing to prevent infusing any more blood. Save the blood tubing and bag for analysis.
• Administer saline solution to keep the vein open.
• Take the patient's vital signs.
• Notify the doctor.
• Obtain urine and blood samples from the patient and send them to the laboratory.
• Prepare for further treatment.
• Complete a transfusion reaction report and an incident report.
Note: The doctor or blood bank may eliminate some of these steps if a patient has had frequent mild reactions.

Transmitted disease. Unlike a transfusion reaction, an infectious disease transmitted during a transfusion may go undetected until days, weeks, or months later, when it produces signs and symptoms. Remember, all blood products are potential carriers of infectious disease, including hepatitis, AIDS, and CMV. Steps to prevent disease transmittal include laboratory testing of blood products and careful screening of potential donors, neither of which is foolproof.
• *Laboratory testing.* Hepatitis C (non-A, non-B) accounts for the majority of posttransfusion hepatitis cases. The test that detects both hepatitis B and hepatitis C can produce false-negative results and may allow some hepatitis to go undetected.

Human immunodeficiency virus (HIV) screening doesn't test specifically for AIDS, but rather for the antibodies to HIV. False-negative results may occur, particularly during the incubation period of about 6 to 12 weeks after exposure. The estimated risk of acquiring HIV from blood products is 1 in 100,000.

Many hospitals screen blood for CMV. Blood with CMV is especially dangerous for an immunosuppressed, seronegative patient. Hospitals also test blood for the presence of syphilis, although the routine practice of refrigerating blood kills the syphilis organism and virtually eliminates the risk of transfusion-related syphilis.

Suggested readings

American Association of Blood Banks. "Blood Transfusion Outside the Hospital," *AJN* 89(4):486-89, April 1989.

Heustis, D.W., et al. *Practical Blood Transfusion,* 4th ed. Boston: Little, Brown & Co., 1988.

Lichtor, J.L. "Transfusion Reactions," Part 2. *Current Reviews for Nurse Anesthetists* 12(4):27-32, July 27, 1989.

7

PARENTERAL NUTRITION

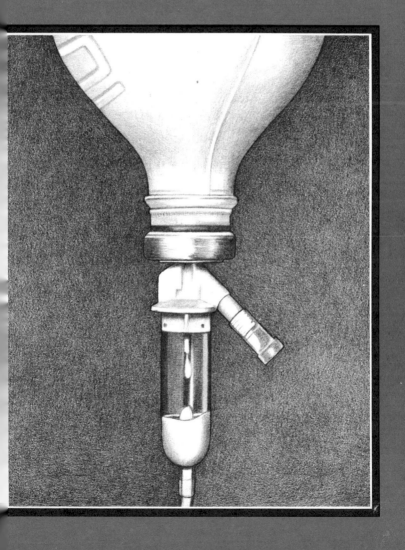

When illness or surgery prevents a patient from eating and metabolizing his food, he may need parenteral nutrition. Depending on the type of therapy ordered, you'll administer nutritional support solutions through either a peripheral or central venous (CV) infusion device. This chapter provides you with the information you need to give parenteral nutrition safely and efficiently by these two methods.

In the first section, you'll review basic nutritional needs, indications for total parenteral nutrition (TPN) and peripheral parenteral nutrition (PPN), and the components of nutritional solutions. This section also explains how to perform a nutritional assessment. In the second section, you'll find information on administering TPN and PPN. And in the last section, you'll review special considerations for pediatric, elderly, and home care patients. This section also tells you which complications to look for and how to discontinue therapy.

Basic concepts

When a nutritional assessment reveals decreased food intake, increased metabolic need, or a combination of both, a doctor may order parenteral nutrition to ensure the patient gets the nutrients he needs. Most patients who require parenteral nutrition therapy receive TPN rather than PPN. Generally, PPN provides fewer nonprotein calories but requires a greater fluid volume for infusion than TPN. Thus, for PPN to deliver the same number of calories as TPN, a much larger volume of fluid must be infused.

Reviewing nutritional needs

Essential nutrients found in food provide energy, maintain body tissues, and aid body processes, such as growth, cell activity, enzyme production, and temperature regulation. Parenteral nutrition solutions can also supply these essential nutrients.

When carbohydrates, lipids, and proteins are metabolized, they produce energy, measured in calories (also called kilocalories). A normal healthy adult requires 2,000 to 3,000 calories/day, depending on his level of physical activity. Any increase in metabolic activity requires an increase in caloric intake. For example, victims of burns, trauma, disease, or stress may require up to 10,000 calories/day.

The most common nutritional deficiencies involve protein and calories. When the body notes these deficiencies, it turns to its reserve sources of energy. Through gluconeogenesis, the body mobilizes and converts glycogen to glucose and urea. Next, the body seeks energy from the fats stored in adipose tissue. As a last resort, the body taps the store of essential visceral and somatic body proteins and converts them to carbohydrates for energy. (Visceral proteins include serum albumin and transferrin. Somatic proteins include skeletal, smooth muscle, and tissue proteins.) When these essential body proteins break down, a catabolic state exists that results in a negative nitrogen balance. Starvation or disease-related stress adds to this catabolic state.

Protein-energy malnutrition. A deficiency of protein and energy (calories) results in protein-energy malnutrition (PEM), also called protein-calorie malnutrition. PEM describes a spectrum of disorders that result from either a prolonged chronic inadequate protein or caloric intake or from high metabolic protein and energy requirements.

Disorders commonly associated with PEM include cancer, GI disorders, chronic heart failure, alcoholism, and conditions causing high metabolic needs, such as burns and infections.

Serious implications of PEM include reduced synthesis of enzymes and plasma proteins; increased susceptibility to infection; physical and mental growth deficiencies in children; severe diarrhea and malabsorption; numerous secondary nutritional deficiencies; delayed wound healing; and mental fatigue.

PEM occurs in three basic forms: iatrogenic PEM, kwashiorkor, and marasmus.

• *Iatrogenic PEM.* Most commonly occurring in patients hospitalized longer than 2 weeks, iatrogenic PEM affects more than 15% of patients in acute care centers. Studies show that during hospitalization a patient's nutritional status often deteriorates, leading to iatrogenic PEM.

• *Kwashiorkor.* Translated literally as *the disease of the deposed baby when the next one is born,* kwashiorkor results from severe protein deficiencies without a caloric deficit and occurs most often in children ages 1 to 3. In the United States, it's usually secondary to malabsorption disorders, cancer and cancer therapies, kidney disease, hypermetabolic illness, and iatrogenic causes.

• *Marasmus.* The third form of malnutrition, marasmus is a prolonged and gradual wasting of muscle mass and subcutaneous fat caused by an inadequate intake of protein, calories, and other nutrients. Marasmus occurs most frequently in infants, ages 6 to 18 months, and in patients with post-gastrectomy dumping syndrome, carcinomas of the mouth and esophagus, and chronic malnutrition states.

Nutritional assessment

To determine if a patient needs parenteral nutrition, you must assess his nutritional status. This includes obtaining a dietary history, performing a physical assessment, making anthropometric measurements, and reviewing the results of pertinent diagnostic tests. Because poor nutritional status can affect most body systems, a thorough nutritional assessment helps you anticipate problems and intervene appropriately.

Dietary history. When obtaining a patient's dietary history, make sure to include the following:
• chief complaint
• present illness
• past medical history, including any previous major illnesses, injuries, hospitalizations, or surgeries
• family history, including any familial, genetic, or environmental illnesses
• social history, including environmental, psychological, and sociological factors that may influence nutritional status, such as living alone or lack of transportation
• dietary recall, using either a 24-hour recall or diet diary
• any factors that may affect food intake.

Physical assessment. Inspect the patient for signs of decreased food intake, increased metabolic requirements, or a combination of the two. Note the presence of poor skin turgor, abnormal pigmentation, hyperpigmentation of the buccal mucosa, exophthalmos, neck swelling, or adventitious lung sounds.

Measuring skin-fold thickness

The two illustrations below show where to place the skin-fold calipers when measuring a patient's triceps and subscapular skin-fold thicknesses.

Triceps skin-fold thickness **Subscapular skin-fold thickness**

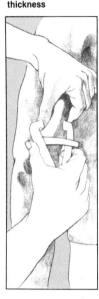 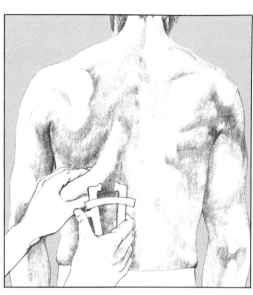

Also note the condition of the patient's teeth or dentures, and look for signs of infection or irritation on the roof of his mouth. Inspect the abdomen for signs of wasting, and palpate for masses, tenderness, and an enlarged liver.

Anthropometry. An objective, noninvasive method of measuring overall body size, composition, and specific body parts, anthropometry compares the patient's measurements with established standards. Commonly used anthropometric measurements include height, weight, ideal body weight, body frame size, skin-fold thickness, midarm circumference, and midarm muscle circumference.

Any finding of less than 90% of the standard measurement may indicate the patient needs nutritional support. (See *Measuring skin-fold thickness.*)

Diagnostic studies. The results of diagnostic studies usually provide the earliest evidence of a nutritional problem. These studies help evaluate visceral protein status, lean body mass, vitamin and mineral balance, and the effectiveness of nutritional support. (See *Detecting nutritional deficiencies with diagnostic tests,* pages 182 and 183.)

Indications for TPN and PPN
A patient may receive TPN for any

of the following reasons:
• debilitating illness lasting longer than 2 weeks
• limited or no oral intake for longer than 7 days, such as in cases of multiple trauma, severe burns, or anorexia nervosa
• at least 10% loss of pre-illness weight
• serum albumin level below 3.5 g/dl
• poor tolerance of long-term enteral feedings
• chronic vomiting or diarrhea
• continued weight loss despite adequate oral intake
• GI disorders that prevent or severely reduce absorption, such as bowel obstruction, Crohn's disease, ulcerative colitis, short bowel syndrome, cancer malabsorption syndrome, and bowel fistulas
• inflammatory GI disorders, such as pancreatitis and peritonitis
• excessive nitrogen loss resulting from wound infection, fistulas, or abscesses
• renal or hepatic failure.

Patients who don't need to gain weight yet need nutritional support may receive PPN for as long as 2 to 3 weeks. It's used to:
• maintain or restore fluid and electrolyte balance and to maintain homeostasis before and after surgery
• help a patient meet minimum calorie and protein requirements.

This therapy may also be used as an adjunct to oral or enteral feedings for a patient needing to supplement his low-calorie intake. Or PPN may be given to a patient who's unable to absorb enteral therapy.

PPN should be used cautiously in patients with severe hepatic damage, coagulation disorders, anemia, and pulmonary disease, and in those at increased risk for fat embolism. It shouldn't be used for patients with malnutrition or fat metabolism disorders, such as pathologic hyperlipidemia, lipid nephrosis, and acute pancreatitis accompanied by hyperlipidemia.

Parenteral nutrition solutions

The specific solution you'll give depends on the type of parenteral nutrition and the patient's status. With some patients, nutritionally incomplete solutions of crystalline amino acids or standard I.V. solutions may be ordered for short-term parenteral nutrition. Special solutions, such as HepatAmine for liver disease and RenAmine for renal disease, may also be prescribed.

Parenteral nutrition solutions consist of the following components, each offering a particular benefit:
• Dextrose. Most calories in parenteral nutrition solutions come from dextrose, which can have a significant nitrogen-sparing effect. The number of nonprotein calories needed to maintain this nitrogen balance depends on the severity of the patient's illness.
• Amino acids. In parenteral nutrition, amino acids supply enough protein to replace essential amino acids, maintain adequate protein stores, and prevent protein loss from muscle tissues.
• Fats. Supplied as lipid emulsions, fats are a concentrated source of energy that prevent or correct fatty acid deficiencies. Available in concentrations of 10% or 20%, lipid emulsions provide 40% to 60% of a patient's daily calories.
• Electrolytes. The number of electrolytes, added to the parenteral nutrition solution, is based on an evaluation of the patient's nutritional needs.
• Vitamins. To ensure normal body functions and optimal utilization of the nutrient substrates, the pa-

Detecting nutritional deficiencies with diagnostic tests

Laboratory studies help pinpoint nutritional deficiencies by aiding in the diagnosis of anemia, malnutrition, and other disorders. The following chart lists some commonly ordered diagnostic tests, their purposes, normal values, and implications.

TEST AND PURPOSE	NORMAL VALUES	IMPLICATIONS
Creatinine height index • Uses a 24-hour urine sample to determine adequacy of muscle mass	• Determined from a reference table of values based on a patient's height or weight	• Less than 80% of reference-standard value: moderate depletion of muscle mass (protein reserves) • Less than 60% of reference-standard value: severe depletion, with increased risk of compromised immune function
Hematocrit • Diagnoses anemia and dehydration	• Male: 42% to 50% • Female: 40% to 48% • Child: 29% to 41% • Neonate: 55% to 68%	• Increased values: severe dehydration, polycythemia • Decreased values: iron-deficiency anemia, excessive blood loss
Hemoglobin • Assesses blood's oxygen-carrying capacity to aid diagnosis of anemia, protein deficiency, and hydration status	• Older adult: 10 to 17 g/dl • Adult male: 13 to 18 g/dl • Adult female: 12 to 16 g/dl • Child: 9.0 to 15.5 g/dl • Neonate: 14 to 20 g/dl	• Increased values: dehydration, polycythemia • Decreased values: protein deficiency, iron-deficiency anemia, excessive blood loss, overhydration
Serum albumin • Helps assess visceral protein stores	• Adult: 3.5 to 5.0 g/dl • Child: same as adult • Neonate: 3.6 to 5.4 g/dl	• Decreased values: malnutrition; liver or kidney disease; congestive heart failure; excessive blood protein losses, such as from severe burns
Serum transferrin (also called serum total iron binding capacity [TIBC]) • Helps assess visceral protein stores; has a shorter half-life than serum albumin and thus more accurately reflects current status	• Adult: 250 to 410 μg/dl • Child: 350 to 450 μg/dl • Neonate: 60 to 175 μg/dl	• Increased TIBC: iron deficiency, as in pregnancy or iron-deficiency anemia • Decreased TIBC: iron excess, as in chronic inflammatory states • Below 200 μg/dl: visceral protein stores depletion • Below 100 μg/dl: severe visceral protein stores depletion
Serum triglycerides • Detects protein-energy malnutrition (PEM) and screens for hyperlipidemia	• 40 to 150 mg/dl	• Increased values combined with increased cholesterol levels: increased risk of atherosclerotic disease • Decreased values: PEM, steatorrhea

Detecting nutritional deficiencies with diagnostic tests *(continued)*

TEST AND PURPOSE	NORMAL VALUES	IMPLICATIONS
Skin sensitivity testing • Evaluates immune response compromised by PEM	• Immunocompetent patients exhibit a positive reaction within 24 hours, marked by a red area of 5 mm or greater at the test site	• Delayed, partial, or negative reaction (no response) may point to PEM
Total lymphocyte count • Diagnoses PEM	• 1,500 to 3,000/mm^3	• Increased values: infection or inflammation, leukemia, tissue necrosis • Decreased values: moderate to severe malnutrition, if no other cause is identified such as influenza or measles
Total protein screen • Detects hyperproteinemia or hypoproteinemia	• 6 to 8 g/dl	• Increased values: dehydration • Decreased values: malnutrition, protein loss
Urine ketone bodies (acetone) • Screens for ketonuria and detects carbohydrate deprivation	• Negative for ketones in urine	• Ketoacidosis starvation

tient needs daily vitamins. A 1-ampule mixture of fat- and water-soluble vitamins, biotin, and folic acid (MVI-12 or MVC 9 + 3) may be added to any single unit of a daily regimen. Imferon may also be added to provide iron.
• Micronutrients. Also called trace elements, micronutrients promote normal metabolism. Commercial solutions contain zinc, copper, chromium, iodide, selenium, and manganese; however, many hospitals mix their own solutions.
• Water. The amount of water added to a parenteral nutrition solution depends on the patient's condition. Retaining fluid balance, considered essential to maintaining the intracellular and extracellular fluid environments, also enhances excretion of metabolites.

Depending on the patient's condition, a doctor may also order additives to the solution, such as insulin or heparin. (For more information, see *Reviewing parenteral therapy solutions*, page 184 and *Understanding common additives*, page 185.)

TPN solutions. Solutions for TPN are hypertonic with an osmolarity of 1,800 to 2,400 mOsm/liter. Electrolytes, vitamins, micronutrients, and water added to the base solution help satisfy daily requirements. Lipids may be given as a separate solution or as a premixed solution with dextrose and amino acids.

Glucose balance is extremely important in a patient receiving TPN. Adults use 0.8 to 1.0 g of glucose

(Text continues on page 186.)

Reviewing parenteral therapy solutions

THERAPY AND SOLUTION	INDICATIONS	SPECIAL CONSIDERATIONS
Total parenteral nutrition • Dextrose, 20% to 25% (1 liter dextrose 25% = 850 nonprotein calories) • Crystalline amino acids, 2.5% to 8.5% • Electrolytes, vitamins, micronutrients, insulin, and heparin as ordered • Fat emulsion, 10% or 20% (usually infused as a separate solution; can be given peripherally or centrally)	Long-term therapy (3 weeks or more) used to: • Supply large quantities of nutrients and calories (2,000 to 2,500 calories/day or more) • Provide needed calories; restore nitrogen balance; replace essential vitamins, electrolytes, minerals, and trace elements • Promote tissue synthesis, wound healing, and normal metabolic function • Allow bowel rest and healing; reduce activity in the gallbladder, pancreas, and small intestine • Improve tolerance to surgery	• Nutritionally complete • Requires minor surgical procedure for central venous (CV) catheter insertion (can be done by the doctor at patient's bedside) • Hypertonic solution • May cause metabolic complications (glucose intolerance, electrolyte imbalances, essential fatty acid deficiency) *I.V. lipid emulsion* • May not be used effectively in severely stressed patients (especially burn patients) • May interfere with immune mechanisms
Peripheral parenteral nutrition • Dextrose, 5% to 10% • Crystalline amino acids, 2.75% to 4.25% • Electrolytes, micronutrients, and vitamins as ordered • Fat emulsion, 10% or 20% (1 liter dextrose 10% and amino acids 3.5% infused at same time with liter lipid emulsion = 1,440 nonprotein calories: 340 from dextrose and 1,100 from lipid emulsion) • Heparin or hydrocortisone as ordered	Short-term therapy (3 weeks or less) used to: • Maintain nutritional state in patients who can tolerate relatively high fluid volume, who usually resume bowel function and oral feedings in a few days, and who are susceptible to catheter-related infections of CV lines • Provide approximately 1,400 to 2,000 calories/day	• Nutritionally complete for short term • Cannot be used in nutritionally depleted patients • Cannot be used in volume-restricted patients since it requires high volumes of solution • Does not cause weight gain • Avoids insertion and maintenance of CV catheter, but patient must have good veins; I.V. site should be changed every 48 hours • Delivers less hypertonic solutions • May cause phlebitis • Less risk of metabolic complications *I.V. lipid emulsion* • As effective as dextrose for caloric source • Diminishes the risk of phlebitis if infused at same time as basic nutrient solution • Irritates vein in long-term use

Understanding common additives

Common components of parenteral nutrition solutions include 50% dextrose in water ($D_{50}W$), amino acids, and any of the additives listed here. These special additives treat a patient's specific metabolic deficiencies.

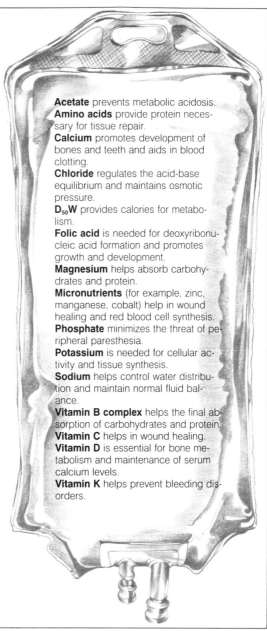

Acetate prevents metabolic acidosis.
Amino acids provide protein necessary for tissue repair.
Calcium promotes development of bones and teeth and aids in blood clotting.
Chloride regulates the acid-base equilibrium and maintains osmotic pressure.
$D_{50}W$ provides calories for metabolism.
Folic acid is needed for deoxyribonucleic acid formation and promotes growth and development.
Magnesium helps absorb carbohydrates and protein.
Micronutrients (for example, zinc, manganese, cobalt) help in wound healing and red blood cell synthesis.
Phosphate minimizes the threat of peripheral paresthesia.
Potassium is needed for cellular activity and tissue synthesis.
Sodium helps control water distribution and maintain normal fluid balance.
Vitamin B complex helps the final absorption of carbohydrates and protein.
Vitamin C helps in wound healing.
Vitamin D is essential for bone metabolism and maintenance of serum calcium levels.
Vitamin K helps prevent bleeding disorders.

Understanding total nutrient admixture

Total nutrient admixture (TNA) is a white solution that delivers 1 day's worth of nutrients in a single 3-liter bag. Also called 3:1 solution, it combines lipids with the other parenteral solution components. Here are answers to some commonly asked questions about TNA.

Who receives TNA?
Only relatively stable patients receive TNA since solution components may be adjusted just once a day.

What are the advantages?
The advantages of TNA include a reduced need to handle the bag, and thus less risk of contamination; decreased nursing time; a reduced need for infusion sets and electronic infusion devices; lower hospital costs; increased patient mobility; and easier adjustment to home care.

What are the disadvantages?
TNA infusion precludes the use of certain infusion pumps because they can't accurately deliver the large volumes of solution. Also, you can't use standard I.V. tubing filters because a 0.22-micron filter won't allow the lipid molecules through.

per kilogram of body weight per hour. That means a patient can tolerate a constant I.V. infusion of a hyperosmolar glucose solution without the addition of exogenous insulin. As the highly concentrated glucose solution infuses, a pancreatic beta-cell response occurs, creating increased serum insulin levels. To allow the pancreas to establish and maintain the necessary increased insulin production, start with a slow infusion rate and increase it gradually. Abrupt cessation

may result in rebound hypoglycemia, so a peripheral infusion of dextrose 10% in water ($D_{10}W$) may be necessary.

Glucose balance may be further compromised by sepsis, stress, shock, hepatic or renal failure, diabetes, age, pancreatic disease, and the concurrent administration of certain medications, including steroids.

Daily allotments of TPN solution, including lipids and other parenteral solution components, can also be administered in a single 3-liter bag (total nutrient admixture). (See *Understanding total nutrient admixture.*)

PPN solutions. Solutions for PPN are nearly isotonic, such as dextrose 5% in water (D_5W), or slightly hypertonic, such as $D_{10}W$ with an osmolarity of 505 mOsm/liter. Lipid emulsions are also given as part of PPN to provide additional calories.

Lipid emulsions. Often infused separately, I.V. lipid emulsions perform exactly the same as digested fat. Cleared from the vascular compartment into storage tissue, they can be oxidized for energy as needed. As a nearly isotonic emulsion, concentrations of both 10% and 20% can be safely infused through peripheral and central veins. Lipid emulsions prevent and treat essential fatty-acid deficiency and provide a major source of energy or an energy-calorie combination.

Essential fatty acids should make up 2% of a patient's daily calories (or up to 10% for a patient with severe deficiency). Some 25% to 40% of TPN calories should be in the form of lipids, while up to 60% of PPN calories may be lipids. A 10% fat emulsion yields 1.1

calorie/ml, and a 20% fat emulsion, 2.2 calories/ml.

Administering parenteral nutrition

Depending on whether the patient needs his nutritional status maintained or replenished, you'll infuse either TPN or PPN. Generally, you'll use TPN to replace nutrients in markedly malnourished and severely catabolic patients to boost their daily caloric intake. (TPN provides 2,000 to 2,500 calories daily.) You'll usually use PPN for maintenance therapy, for patients who've had nothing by mouth for more than 3 days, and for those who aren't expected to eat again for the next 10 to 14 days. (PPN supplies 1,400 to 2,000 calories daily.)

You'll deliver the parenteral nutrition either continuously or cyclically. With continuous parenteral nutrition, the patient receives the infusion over a 24-hour period. The infusion begins at a slow rate and gradually increases to the rate ordered by the doctor. This treatment helps avoid complications, such as rebound hypoglycemia, frequently associated with other methods.

A patient undergoing cyclic therapy receives 1,000 to 2,000 parenteral calories overnight and the balance of his nutrients orally the next day. Home care parenteral nutrition programs have boosted the popularity of cyclic therapy, which may also be used to wean the patient from TPN.

When switching from continuous to cyclic TPN, adjust the flow rate so the patient's blood glucose level can adapt to the new therapy. Do this by reducing the flow rate by one half for 1 hour before stopping the continuous infusion. Draw a blood glucose sample 1 hour into the new schedule and observe the patient for hypoglycemic signs during the first 2 hours.

Administering TPN
TPN solutions must be infused in a central vein, using either a peripherally inserted catheter whose tip lies in a central vein, a CV catheter, or an implanted vascular access device. Long-term therapy requires either a Silastic CV catheter, such as a Hickman, Broviac, or Groshong catheter, or an implanted vascular access device, such as the Infuse-A-Port or Port-A-Cath.

Because TPN fluid has about six times the solute concentration of blood, peripheral I.V. administration results in sclerosis and thrombosis. To ensure optimal dilution, the CV catheter should be in the superior vena cava — a wide-bore, high-flow vein. Usually, the catheter isn't advanced into the right atrium because of the risk of cardiac perforation and arrhythmias.

Preparing the patient. To increase compliance, make sure your patient understands the purpose of his treatment, and enlist his help throughout the course of therapy. Understanding TPN and its goals also helps a home care patient assume a greater role in administering, monitoring, documenting, and maintaining his therapy.

Focus your teaching on the signs and symptoms that accompany fluid, electrolyte, and glucose imbalances, as well as vitamin and trace element deficiencies and toxicities. To avoid glucose imbalance, teach the patient to regulate the flow rate and stress

Precautions for giving lipid emulsions

You may administer lipid emulsions as part of a total parenteral nutrition solution, along with a peripheral parenteral nutrition solution, or separately through either a central venous or a peripheral line. No matter which of these methods you use, be sure you observe these precautions:
☐ Use a particulate filter according to the manufacturer's recommendations (a 1.2-micron filter is preferred). Standard 0.22-micron filters are insufficient because lipid particles clot the filter and disturb the emulsion.
☐ Before the infusion, always check the lipid emulsion for separation or an oily appearance. If either condition exists, the lipid may have been disturbed and shouldn't be used. Never shake the lipid container excessively or use the emulsion if any inconsistency in texture or color appears.
☐ Never add anything to the lipid emulsion; doing so could cause instability. Also, protect the emulsion from freezing.
☐ Discard any unused portion; a contaminated emulsion can support microbial growth. The Centers for Disease Control guidelines recommend not hanging lipid emulsions longer than 12 hours. Follow the manufacturer's recommendations.
☐ During the initial lipid infusion, monitor the patient's vital signs. The flow rate shouldn't exceed 1 ml/minute for the first 30 minutes.
☐ Check for signs and symptoms of a reaction. Indications of an immediate reaction, which can occur within 2½ hours, include increased temperature, flushing, sweating, pressure sensations over the eyes, nausea, vomiting, headache, chest and back pain, dyspnea, and cyanosis. Indications of a delayed reaction, which occur up to 10 days after the infusion, include hepatomegaly, splenomegaly, thrombocytopenia, focal seizures, hyperlipidemia, hepatic damage, jaundice, hemorrhagic diathesis, and gastroduodenal ulcer.
☐ Be aware of the biochemical and clinical signs and symptoms of essential fatty acid disease that may be associated with impaired wound healing, adverse effects on red blood cells, and ineffective prostaglandin synthesis. Check for dry or scaly skin, thinning hair, liver function abnormalities, and thrombocytopenia.

the importance of maintaining that rate. Explain that a gradual increase in flow rate, approximately 25 ml/hour per day, allows the pancreas to establish and maintain the increased insulin production necessary to tolerate this treatment.

Describe the administration schedule. And to avoid incompatibilities, review prescribed and over-the-counter medications the patient now takes. Finally, familiarize the patient with the equipment that will be used.

Preparing the equipment. Before TPN administration can begin, a doctor must insert a CV access device—either a CV catheter or an implanted vascular device. To administer TPN, you need to gather the TPN solution, a controller or pump, a nonphthalate administration set, alcohol swabs, and an I.V. pole.

Because the infusion of a chilled solution can cause pain, hypothermia, venous spasm, and venous constriction, be sure to remove a 1-liter bag or bottle of TPN solution from the refrigerator 30 minutes before use. Plan to remove a 2- or 3-liter bag 6 to 8 hours before use.

If the TPN solution contains lipid emulsions, you'll have to take special precautions. (See *Precautions for giving lipid emulsions.*)

Initiating the infusion. Begin the infusion at a slow rate (usually 40 ml/hour), as ordered, to reduce the risk of hyperglycemia. Then, increase the infusion rate as ordered (usually in 25 ml/hour increments). In adults, this rate allows the pancreatic beta cells to increase endogenous insulin production and to establish carbohydrate and water tolerance.

Watch for swelling at the catheter insertion site. This may indicate extravasation of the TPN solution, which can cause necrosis.

Always maintain strict aseptic technique when handling the equipment used to administer therapy. Because the TPN solution serves as a medium for bacterial growth and the CV line provides systemic access, the patient risks infection and sepsis.

When using a filter, position it as close to the access site as possible. Check the filter's porosity and psi capacity to make sure it exceeds the psi exerted by the positive-pressure pump.

Maintaining the infusion. Carefully monitor the patient and assess his response to the therapy to detect early signs of metabolic complications such as hyperglycemia or hypocalcemia. If you spot a problem, notify the doctor so the TPN regimen can be changed.

If the patient tolerates the solution well the first day, the doctor will usually increase the intake to 1 liter every 12 hours for at least 2 days. After the first 3 to 5 days of TPN, most patients can tolerate 3 liters of solution per day without adverse effects.

To maintain a TPN infusion, remember these key points:
• Make sure each bag or bottle has a label listing the expiration date, time the solution was hung, glucose concentration, and total volume of solution. (If the bag or bottle is damaged and you don't have an immediate replacement, you can approximate the glucose concentration until the new container is ready by adding 50% glucose to $D_{10}W$.)
• Don't allow TPN solutions to hang for more than 24 hours.
• Maintain flow rates as prescribed, even if the flow falls behind schedule.
• Expect to change the tubing and filter every 24 hours, using strict aseptic technique. Make sure all tubing junctions are secure.
• Perform I.V. site care and dressing changes at least three times a week (once a week for transparent semi-permeable dressings), or whenever the dressing becomes wet, nonocclusive, or soiled. Use strict aseptic technique.
• Check the infusion pump's volume meter and time tape every 30 minutes (or more often, if necessary) to avoid an irregular flow rate.
• Record vital signs every 4 to 8 hours (or more often, if necessary). Be alert for increased temperature—one of the earliest signs of catheter-related sepsis.
• Collect a double-voided urine specimen every 6 hours and test for glucose and acetone. Notify the doctor if you observe glycosuria. If glycosuria persists, anticipate fingerstick blood glucose testing.
• Be careful when using the TPN infusion line for other functions. If using a single-lumen CV catheter,

don't use the line to infuse blood or blood products, to give a bolus injection, to administer simultaneous I.V. solutions, to measure CV pressure, or to draw blood for laboratory tests. Remember, never add medication to a TPN solution container. Also, don't use a three-way stopcock if possible; add-on devices increase the risk of infection.

• Accurately record the patient's daily fluid intake and output, specifying the volume and type of each fluid, and calculate the daily caloric intake. This record serves as a diagnostic tool for prompt, precise replacement of fluid and electrolyte deficits.

• Assess the patient's physical status daily. Weigh him at the same time each morning (after voiding), in similar clothing, using the same scale. Suspect fluid imbalance if the patient gains more than 1.1 lb (0.5 kg)/day. If ordered, measure arm circumference, triceps, and skin-fold thickness.

• Monitor the results of routine laboratory tests, such as serum electrolytes, blood urea nitrogen, and glucose, and report abnormal findings to the doctor so appropriate changes in the TPN solution can be made.

• Monitor the patient for signs and symptoms of nutritional aberrations, such as fluid and electrolyte imbalances and glucose metabolism disturbances. Some patients may require supplementary insulin for the duration of TPN; the pharmacy usually adds this directly to the TPN solution.

• Provide emotional support. Keep in mind that patients often associate eating with positive feelings and become disturbed when it's eliminated.

• Provide frequent mouth care for the patient.

• Document all assessment findings and nursing interventions.

Administering PPN

Using a combination of amino acid-dextrose solution and lipid emulsion, PPN supplies the patient's full caloric needs without the risks associated with central vein access. Because a PPN solution has a lower tonicity than a TPN solution, a patient receiving PPN must be able to tolerate the large volumes of fluid.

Preparing the patient. Make sure the patient understands what to expect before, during, and after therapy.

Select the patient's largest available vein as the insertion site to provide hemodilution of the irritating PPN solution. When using a short-term catheter that requires 48- to 72-hour site rotation, try applying heat to the site to facilitate insertion.

Preparing the equipment. To administer PPN, you need an amino acid-dextrose solution (at room temperature), lipid emulsion, two controllers or pumps, a Y-type nonphthalate administration set, alcohol swabs, and an I.V. pole. You may also need venipuncture equipment.

When administering lipids and amino acids together, use the Y-type nonphthalate administration set to avoid having lipids extract small amounts of phthalates from polyvinylchloride tubing. Use a vented line for the lipid emulsion; use a filtered line for the amino acid-dextrose solution. Hang the lipid emulsion container higher than the amino acid-dextrose container so the lipid emulsion doesn't backflow into the amino acid set. (See *Giving lipids and amino acids together.*)

To ensure the correct infusion

rate, use controllers that can accommodate the special tubing. Remember, the risk of phlebitis decreases when you administer two components at about the same rate.

Initiating the infusion. To initiate PPN, follow these steps:
• Inspect the lipid emulsion for opacity and consistency of color and texture. If it looks frothy or oily, if it contains particles, or if you question its stability or sterility, return the bottle to the pharmacy. Avoid shaking the bottle excessively to help prevent aggregation of fat globules.
• Similarly, inspect the amino acid-dextrose solution for cloudiness, turbidity, and particles and the bottle for cracks; if any of these exist, return the bottle to the pharmacy.
• Wash your hands and, using aseptic technique, take the nonphthalate tubing from its package. Close the flow clamp to equalize pressure in the tubing.
• Remove the protective cap from the lipid emulsion bottle and wipe the rubber stopper with an alcohol swab. Hold the bottle upright and insert the vented spike through the inner circle of the rubber stopper. Hang the bottle, and squeeze the drip chamber until it fills to the level indicated in the tubing instructions. Open the flow clamp, allow the emulsion to flow through to the Y-connector, and close the clamp.
• Remove the protective cap from the container of amino acid-dextrose solution, and wipe the rubber stopper with an alcohol swab. Hold the bottle upright, and insert the spike. Hang the bottle, and squeeze the drip chamber until the fluid reaches the desired level. Hold the filter with the Y-connector facing upward. Open the clamp and let the

Giving lipids and amino acids together

The illustration below shows the setup you'll use to administer lipid emulsions with amino acids. Note that the lipid emulsion container is higher than the amino acid container.

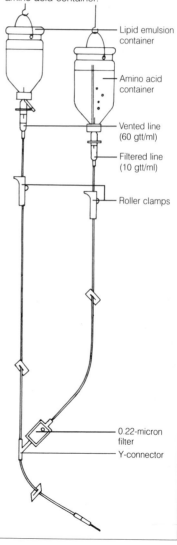

- Lipid emulsion container
- Amino acid container
- Vented line (60 gtt/ml)
- Filtered line (10 gtt/ml)
- Roller clamps
- 0.22-micron filter
- Y-connector

solution flow until the filter and line are free of air. If your set contains a second Y-site, invert it and tap gently to remove all the air from the tubing. Close the clamp.
• Then, attach the pumps or controllers to the I.V. pole, and prepare them according to the manufacturer's instructions.
• If necessary, perform a venipuncture and then connect the administration set to the I.V. needle or catheter hub. Turn on the controllers and set them to the ordered flow rate. It should start slowly and gradually increase to ensure tolerance to the hypertonic solution, $D_{10}W$ glucose solution, if used. Next, completely open the flow clamps and let the controllers regulate the flow rate.
• Monitor the patient's vital signs every 10 minutes for the first 30 minutes, and every hour thereafter.

Maintaining the infusion. Caring for a patient receiving a PPN infusion involves the same steps you'd take for any patient receiving a peripheral I.V. infusion, including maintaining the solution, tubing, dressings, site, and I.V. devices. To maintain the infusion, keep these guidelines in mind:
• Monitor the patient for signs of sepsis, such as elevated temperature, glycosuria, chills, malaise, leukocytosis, and altered level of consciousness.
• Observe the patient's reaction to the lipid emulsion. Patients commonly report a feeling of satiety; occasionally, they complain of an unpleasant metallic taste.
• Check the lipid emulsion clearance rate. Lipid emulsion may clear from the blood at an accelerated rate in a patient with full-thickness burns, multiple trauma, or metabolic imbalance because catecholamines, adre-

nocortical hormones, thyroxine, and growth hormone enhance lipolysis and mobilization of fatty acids.
• Check serum triglyceride levels; these should return to normal within 18 hours after lipid emulsion infusion. Typically, alanine aminotransferase (ALT, formerly SGPT), aspartate aminotransferase (AST, formerly SGOT), alkaline phosphatase, cholesterol, triglyceride, plasma-free fatty acid, and coagulation tests are performed weekly.
• Because lipase synthesis increases insulin requirements, expect to increase the insulin dosage of a diabetic patient, as ordered. For a patient with hypothyroidism, administer thyroid-stimulating hormone, as ordered, to affect lipase activity and to prevent intravascular accumulations of triglycerides.
• Monitor for immediate or early adverse reactions to lipid emulsion therapy. Occurring in fewer than 1% of patients, these reactions may include fever, dyspnea, cyanosis, nausea, vomiting, headache, flushing, diaphoresis, lethargy, syncope, chest and back pain, slight pressure over the eyes, irritation at the infusion site, hyperlipemia, hypercoagulability, and thrombocytopenia.

Precautions and complications

If you're administering parenteral nutrition to a pediatric or elderly patient or if you're caring for a patient who'll be receiving therapy at home, you need to be aware of some special considerations. Also, during therapy for any patient, you must monitor for complications, such as air embolism. Finally, you need to know how to discontinue therapy safely and correctly.

Patients with special needs

Pediatric, elderly, and home care patients all have special nursing needs. With pediatric and elderly patients, for instance, you must be particularly careful to administer the correct volume of parenteral nutrition solution. When you're caring for a patient who'll continue therapy at home, you'll need to teach him the appropriate procedures and precautions.

Pediatric patients. Parenteral feedings must not only maintain a child's nutritional status but also fuel his growth. Overall, a child has a greater need for protein, carbohydrates, fat, electrolytes, micronutrients, vitamins, and fluid than an adult. This increased need makes the accurate calculation of solution components and formulations imperative.

Be aware that the child's age, activity level, maturity, size, development, and psychosocial status may affect the outcome of therapy. Also, recognize that administration of PPN with lipid emulsions in a premature or low birth-weight infant may cause lipid accumulation in the lungs. Thrombocytopenia has also been reported in infants receiving 20% lipid emulsions.

Elderly patients. Overinfusion in an elderly patient can produce serious effects, so always monitor flow rates carefully. Also, an elderly patient may be confused or have underlying clinical problems that affect the outcome of his treatment. For example, he may be taking medications that can interact with the components in the parenteral nutrition solution. For this reason, ask the pharmacist about possible interactions with any drug the patient is taking.

Home care patients. Giving parenteral nutrition therapy at home has dramatically improved the health of patients with chronic conditions, such as Crohn's disease and malabsorption syndrome; patients with acute conditions, such as incomplete bowel obstruction; and those receiving antineoplastic therapy. Although PPN therapy may be administered at home, long-term TPN is the primary home care therapy.

If your patient will be receiving parenteral nutrition at home, you'll need to teach him and his family or other caregiver how to administer the therapy and manage complications.

Assess the patient's ability to perform the necessary routine care. Consider his motivation, mental aptitude, work schedule, daily activities, home environment, and accessibility to hospitals or other health care support systems. Determine if his family members or friends can assist him, if necessary.

Establish a suitable schedule with the patient, taking into consideration his nutritional needs as well as his life-style. Stress the importance of adhering to this schedule to prevent glucose imbalance. Record his learning progress in the nurses' notes.

• *Patient teaching.* Teach your patient the procedures for administering therapy (including the use of pumps or controllers), for disposing of supplies, and for measuring urine glucose. Instruct him to change his dressing as directed, or whenever it becomes soiled, wet, or nonocclusive, and to change the

(Text continues on page 196.)

COMPLICATIONS

 Dealing with TPN hazards

Complications of total parenteral nutrition (TPN) therapy can result from catheter-related, metabolic, or mechanical problems. To help you identify and treat these common complications, use this chart.

COMPLICATIONS	SIGNS AND SYMPTOMS	INTERVENTIONS
Catheter-related complications		
Dislodged catheter	Catheter out of the vein	• Place a sterile gauze pad on the insertion site and apply pressure.
Cracked or broken tubing	Fluid leaking out of the tubing	• Apply a padded hemostat above the break to prevent air from entering the line.
Pneumothorax and hydrothorax	Dyspnea, chest pain, cyanosis, decreased breath sounds	• Suction. • Chest tube will be inserted.
Sepsis	Fever, chills, leukocytosis, erythema or pus at insertion site	• Remove catheter and culture tip. • Give appropriate antibiotics.
Metabolic complications		
Hyperglycemia	Fatigue, restlessness, confusion, anxiety, weakness, and (in severe cases) delirium or coma; polyuria; dehydration; elevated blood and urine glucose levels	• Start insulin therapy or adjust TPN flow rate.
Hypoglycemia	Sweating, shaking, irritability when infusion is stopped	• Infuse dextrose 10%.
Hyperosmolar non-ketotic syndrome	Confusion, lethargy, seizures, coma, hyperglycemia, dehydration, glycosuria	• Stop dextrose. • Give insulin and 0.45% sodium chloride to rehydrate.
Hypokalemia	Muscle weakness, paralysis, paresthesia, arrhythmias	• Increase potassium supplementation.
Hypomagnesemia	Tingling around mouth, paresthesia in fingers, mental changes, hyperreflexia	• Increase magnesium supplementation.
Hypophosphatemia	Irritability, weakness, paresthesia, coma, respiratory arrest	• Increase phosphate supplementation.

COMPLICATIONS

 Dealing with TPN hazards *(continued)*

COMPLICATIONS	SIGNS AND SYMPTOMS	INTERVENTIONS
Hypocalcemia	Polyuria, dehydration, elevated blood and urine glucose levels	• Increase calcium supplementation.
Metabolic acidosis	Increased serum chloride level, decreased serum bicarbonate level	• Use acetate or lactate salts of sodium or hydrogen.
Hepatic dysfunction	Increased serum transaminase, lactate dehydrogenase, and bilirubin levels	• Use special hepatic formulations. • Decrease carbohydrate and add I.V. lipids.
Mechanical complications		
Clotted catheter	Interrupted flow rate, hypoglycemia	• Reposition catheter. Attempt to aspirate clot. • If·unsuccessful, instill urokinase to clear catheter lumen, as ordered.
Air embolism	Apprehension, chest pain, tachycardia, hypotension, cyanosis, seizure, loss of consciousness, cardiac arrest	• Clamp catheter. • Place patient in the Trendelenburg position on left side. • Give oxygen as ordered. • If cardiac arrest occurs, use cardiopulmonary resuscitation.
Thrombosis	Erythema and edema at insertion site; ipsilateral swelling of arm, neck, and face; pain at the insertion site and along vein; malaise; fever; tachycardia	• Remove catheter promptly. • Administer heparin, if ordered. • Venous flow studies may be done.
Too rapid an infusion	Nausea, headache, lethargy	• Check the infusion rate. • Check the infusion pump if you're using one.
Extravasation	Swelling of tissue around the insertion site; pain	• Stop I.V. infusion. • Assess patient for cardiopulmonary abnormalities. Chest X-ray may be performed.
Phlebitis	Pain, tenderness, redness, and warmth	• Apply gentle heat to the insertion site. • Elevate the insertion site, if possible.

tubing as scheduled. Remind him not to let the catheter come in contact with granular or lint-producing surfaces to avoid a local tissue reaction.

Explain to the patient that after the catheter has been in place at least 1 month, the doctor may allow him to remove the dressing to bathe or shower. If the patient will be using a pump or controller, mention that he may need a three-prong adapter for his household electrical outlets.

Also discuss outside services that offer help and advice for home care patients, such as hospitals, and philanthropic organizations that provide financial support for this extremely expensive therapy. Tell an elderly patient that Medicare may assume the cost of supplies and parenteral solutions if he meets eligibility requirements.

Although a nurse from the home health care team should always be available to the patient, suggest that he wear a Medic-Alert bracelet or subscribe to a medical alert service.

Explain the complications the patient faces and how he should handle them.
• *Making arrangements.* Upon discharge, arrange for a follow-up physical examination and laboratory work. You may also be asked to arrange for a home care agency to help the patient adjust to therapy and resolve any difficulties. Finally, give the patient the supplies he needs — including dressings, tubing, and TPN solution — and tell him how to get more supplies.

A long-term parenteral nutrition patient needs the help of a home care nurse. She can help his transition to home care by meeting with him in the hospital and making sure the pump he's using in the hospital is the same pump he'll be using at home.

Complications

Patients receiving parenteral nutrition therapy face many of the same complications as patients undergoing any peripheral I.V. or CV therapy. TPN and PPN also pose their own distinct risks.

Complications of TPN therapy may result from catheter-related, metabolic, or mechanical problems. Sepsis, the most serious catheter-related complication, can be fatal; fortunately, you can prevent it with meticulous, consistent catheter care. The most common metabolic complications include hyperglycemia, hypokalemia, and hypomagnesemia. Common mechanical complications include catheter lumen obstruction, air embolism, thrombosis, and extravasation. (See *Dealing with TPN hazards,* pages 194 and 195.)

Common complications of PPN therapy include phlebitis and extravasation.

Prolonged administration of lipid emulsion can produce delayed complications, including hepatomegaly, splenomegaly, jaundice secondary to central lobular cholestasis, blood dyscrasias (thrombocytopenia and leukopenia), and transient increases in liver function studies. A small number of patients receiving 20% I.V. lipid emulsion develop brown pigmentation (I.V. fat pigment in the reticuloendothelial system).

Discontinuing therapy

You'll follow the same basic procedure when discontinuing TPN and PPN therapy — with one major difference. A patient receiving TPN must be weaned from therapy — and then, only if he's receiving some other form of nutritional therapy, such as oral feedings. A patient receiving PPN can discontinue therapy without being weaned. Often, such a patient is only undergoing a solution change, for example, $D_{10}W$ to D_5W.

When discontinuing TPN therapy, you'll wean the patient over 24 to 48 hours to prevent rebound hypoglycemia. The doctor will probably decrease the solution amount by 1 liter/day, and sometimes a solution of $D_{10}W$ may be used to help wean the patient.

During this process, decrease the infusion rate slowly, depending on the patient's current glucose intake. Use a cyclic administration schedule to wean a patient from TPN to enteral feedings.

Suggested readings

Delaney, C.W., and Lauer, M.L. *Intravenous Therapy: A Guide to Quality Care.* Philadelphia: J.B. Lippincott Co., 1988.

Grimble G., and Silk, D. "Administration of Fat Emulsions with Nutritional Mixtures from the 3-liter Delivery System in TPN: Efficacy and Safety," *Nutritional Support Services* 7(10):14-16, 391, October 1987.

Jeppsson, R.I. "Compatibility of Parenteral Nutrition Solutions When Mixed in EVA Plastic Bags," *Nutritional Support Services* 7(10):16, 21, October 1987.

Plumer A. *Principles and Practice of Intravenous Therapy,* 4th ed. Boston: Little, Brown & Co., 1987.

SELF-TEST

Test your I.V. therapy knowledge and skills at your own pace by answering the multiple-choice questions on pages 199 to 201. Questions may have more than one correct answer. Answers appear on page 201.

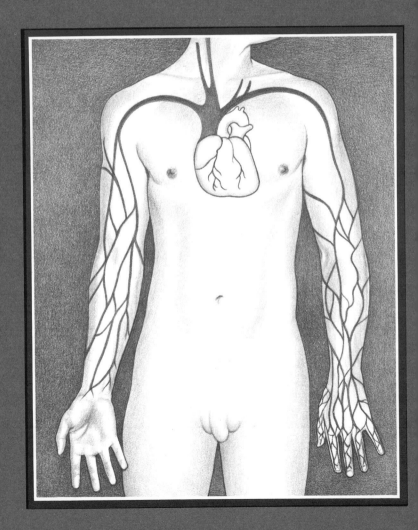

1. *Which of the following is* not *a purpose of I.V. therapy?*
a. to provide enteral nutrition
b. to maintain fluid and electrolyte balance
c. to provide parenteral nutrition
d. to administer medications

2. *Which type of solution raises serum osmolarity and pulls fluid and electrolytes from the intracellular and the intrastitial compartments into the intravascular compartment?*
a. isotonic
b. hypertonic
c. electrotonic
d. hypotonic

3. *The term homeostasis describes:*
a. fluid balance.
b. electrolyte movement.
c. action of water in the body.
d. the maintenance of urine output.

4. *All of the following affect I.V. flow rates* except:
a. fluid viscosity.
b. length of the venipuncture device.
c. container height.
d. gauge of the venipuncture device.

5. *Which precautions should you use to prevent intravascular infections?*
a. Tape the venipuncture device securely to prevent motion.
b. Change insertion sites according to hospital policy.
c. Apply the tourniquet 6" to 8" (14.4 to 20.3 cm) above the insertion site.
d. After an unsuccessful venipuncture, remove the device and reinsert it into another vein.

6. *Which techniques should you use to distend veins?*
a. Apply the tourniquet tight enough to trap venous blood.
b. Hold the patient's hand above his head for 2 minutes.
c. Have the patient make a tight fist several times.
d. Apply cold packs.

7. *Which of the following statements are true?*
a. An absence of blood return indicates infiltration.
b. If an I.V. infusion runs dry, a blood clot may form in the venipuncture device.
c. A vesicant drug can cause tissue necrosis.
d. You should secure the venipuncture device by placing tape around the entire arm.

8. *When positioned properly, the tip of a central venous (CV) catheter should lie in the:*
a. superior vena cava.
b. basilic vein.
c. jugular vein.
d. subclavian vein.

9. *If a CV catheter becomes disconnected accidently, you should immediately:*
a. call the doctor.
b. apply a dry sterile dressing to the site.
c. clamp the catheter.
d. tell the patient to take a deep breath and hold it.

10. *When a CV catheter dressing becomes moist or loose, you should first:*
a. draw a circle around the moist spot and note the date and time.
b. notify the doctor.
c. remove the catheter, check for catheter integrity, and send the tip for culture.
d. remove the dressing, clean the site, and apply a new dressing.

11. *The Valsalva maneuver:*
a. may prove too difficult for patients to learn.
b. can be used anytime the catheter is open to air.
c. helps the doctor locate landmarks more readily during catheter insertion.
d. helps stabilize the catheter during suturing.

12. *Implanted vascular access ports (VAPs) are:*
a. safe and effective means of delivering all types of I.V. drugs and solutions.

b. frequently used in outpatients.
c. indicated for patients who periodically need I.V. access (for chemotherapy or blood administration, for example).
d. all of the above.

13. *What type of needle would you use to access a VAP?*
a. hypodermic needle
b. non-coring needle
c. spinal needle
d. 16G needle

14. *If you meet resistance while trying to flush a VAP, you should:*
a. use a 1-ml syringe filled with heparin solution to briskly flush the device.
b. immediately call the doctor so he can flush the device.
c. stop trying to flush the device, ask the patient to turn on his side or raise his arms, then slowly reattempt to flush.
d. ask the doctor to consult a surgeon about removing the device.

15. *Volume-control sets are recommended for infants and small children because they:*
a. limit the volume available to the child.
b. provide a way of administering a small volume of a drug intermittently.
c. decrease the risk of inadvertent fluid overload.
d. all of the above.

16. *The most common drug administration error is:*
a. mixing incompatible drugs.
b. administering an incorrect dosage.
c. failing to positively identify the patient.
d. using an incorrect administration method.

17. *Donor blood is routinely tested for all of the following* except:
a. syphilis.
b. HLA compatibility.
c. general antibodies.
d. hepatitis B.

18. *The maximum transfusion time for a unit of packed red blood cells is:*
a. 6 hours.
b. 4 hours.
c. 2 hours.
d. 1 hour.

19. *A key requirement for a blood transfusion in the home is that:*
a. the patient's identification band appear on the unit of blood and return with the empty blood bag.
b. premedications be routinely used to reduce the risk of transfusion reactions.
c. a standing order exist for emergency drugs, which must be available.
d. a family member be present for 2 hours after the transfusion.

20. *Which is the most common type of immediate transfusion reaction?*
a. hemolytic
b. febrile
c. allergic
d. bacterial

21. *Potential complications of a massive transfusion include:*
a. alkalosis.
b. increased 2,3-DPG and hyperthermia.
c. hypocalcemia and hyperkalemia.
d. elevated leukocyte count and hemodilution.

22. *Why should you start a blood transfusion at a slow rate?*
a. to prevent clot formation at the tip of the venipuncture device
b. to prevent blood leakage at the insertion site
c. to minimize the effect of any transfusion reaction
d. to allow saline solution enough time to dilute the blood

23. *The major source of calories in parenteral nutrition comes from:*
a. dextrose.
b. amino acids.
c. lipids.
d. vitamins.

24. *Which of these commonly used anthropometric measurements help determine nutritional status?*
a. weight
b. midarm muscle circumference
c. triceps skinfold measurement
d. all of the above

25. *Which of these is a sign of an immediate adverse reaction to lipid emulsion administration?*
a. rock-hard eyes
b. jaundice
c. temperature drop
d. splenomegaly

26. *Which of the following should you teach a patient who'll be receiving total parenteral nutrition at home?*
a. how to use the electronic flow controller
b. how to maintain the catheter
c. how to recognize complications
d. all of the above

ANSWERS

1. a	**6.** a, c	**11.** b	**16.** c	**21.** c
2. b	**7.** b, c	**12.** d	**17.** b	**22.** c
3. a	**8.** a	**13.** b	**18.** b	**23.** a
4. b	**9.** c	**14.** c	**19.** c	**24.** d
5. a, b	**10.** d	**15.** d	**20.** b	**25.** a
				26. d

APPENDICES
AND
INDEX

COMMON ABBREVIATIONS

AA	amino acids
b.i.d.	twice daily (while awake)
D	dextrose solution
D$_5$LR	dextrose 5% in Ringer's injection, lactated
D$_5$R	dextrose 5% in Ringer's injection
D-S	dextrose-saline combinations
D$_{2.5}$½NS or D$_{2.5}$½NaCl	dextrose 2.5% in sodium chloride 0.45%
D$_{2.5}$NS or D$_{2.5}$NaCl	dextrose 2.5% in sodium chloride 0.9%
D$_5$¼NS or D$_5$0.2 NaCl	dextrose 5% in sodium chloride 0.225%
D$_5$½NS or D$_5$0.45 NaCl	dextrose 5% in sodium chloride 0.45%
D$_5$NS or D$_5$0.9 NaCl	dextrose 5% in sodium chloride 0.9%
D$_{10}$NS or D$_{10}$0.9 NaCl	dextrose 10% in sodium chloride 0.9%
D$_5$W	dextrose 5% in water
D$_{10}$W	dextrose 10% in water
DXN-NS	dextran 6% in sodium chloride 0.9%
g	gram
G	gauge
gr	grain
gtt	drop
h or hr	hour
h.s.	at bedtime
IS	invert sugar
kg	kilogram
L or l	liter
LR or RL	Ringer's injection, lactated
mcg or μg	microgram
mEq	milliequivalent
mg	milligram
ml	milliliter
mm	millimeter
N.P.O.	nothing by mouth
NS or NSS	sodium chloride 0.9%
P.O.	by mouth
p.r.n.	as needed
pt	pint
q	every
q.d.	every day
q.h.	every hour
q.i.d.	four times daily (while awake)
R	Ringer's injection
RBC	red blood cell
stat	immediately
t.i.d.	three times daily (while awake)
TPN	total parenteral nutrition
U	unit
W	sterile water for injection
WBC	white blood cell

I.V. DRUG COMPATIBILITY

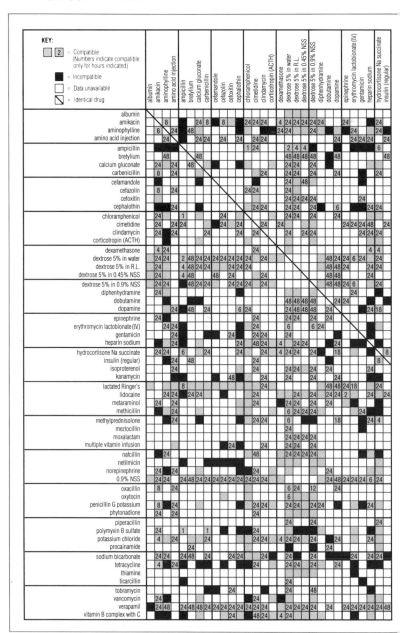

	isoproterenol	kanamycin	lactated Ringer's	lidocaine	metaraminol	methicillin	methylprednisolone	mezlocillin	moxalactam	multiple vitamin infusion	nafcillin	netilmicin	norepinephrine	0.9% NSS	oxytocin	penicillin G potassium	phytonadione	piperacillin	polymyxin B sulfate	potassium chloride	procainamide	sodium bicarbonate	tetracycline	thiamine	ticarcillin	tobramycin	vancomycin	verapamil	vitamin B complex with C
albumin					24									24	24	8		8	24		24	4		24	4			24	24
amikacin			24								24			24									24						48
aminophylline	24		24	24	24	24					24		24			24		24	24		24		24						
amino acid injection		8								24			24				1							24				24	
ampicillin			24								48									24	48							48	
bretylium			24								24																	48	
carbenicillin											24						1	24		24								24	
calcium gluconate											24																	24	
cefamandole											24																	24	
cefazolin	48							24			24									24				24		24	24		
cefoxitin											24									24								24	
cephalothin											24																	24	
chloramphenicol	24		24	24		24			48		24	24			24	24		24	24		24				24	24	48		
cimetidine	24	24			24		24				24			24	24		24		24		24				24	24			
clindamycin									4																			4	
corticotropin (ACTH)	24	24		24	6	6	24	24	24	24			6	6	24		24		24	24		24	24		24	24	24		
dexamethasone	24		24	24	24			24	24	24			24	24														24	
dextrose 5% in water			24	24	24			24	24							12		24		24		24	24		48			24	
dextrose 5% in R.L.													24															24	
dextrose 5% in 0.45% NSS	24		48	24	24								24	24							24							24	
dextrose 5% in 0.9% NSS	24	48	24		18								48	24						24			24					24	
diphenhydramine			24	2									24															24	
dobutamine			18										24								24							24	
dopamine					24								24															24	
epinephrine	24		24			24							6		24					24		24						24	
erythromycin lactobionate (IV)			24			4							24					24		24								24	
gentamicin			24																									48	
heparin sodium			24										24															24	
hydrocortisone Na succinate			24										24															24	
insulin (regular)	24	24		24		24			24	24	24				8		24		24		24	24	24	24		24	48	24	24	24
isoproterenol			24															24							24	24			48
kanamycin			24													6								24					24
lactated Ringer's		24														6													24
lidocaine			24			24			4			24 24	24					24		4				24 24					24
metaraminol		24														24						24							24
methicillin			24							24																			24
methylprednisolone						24																24							24
mezlocillin	24 24		24		24	6		6	24	24	24				8		24		24		24	24	24	24		24	48	24	24
moxalactam		24													8														24
multiple vitamin infusion		24			24			24		4				24								24							24
nafcillin		24																				24							24
netilmicin			24											24															
norepinephrine	24 24		24		24	6		6	24	24	24				8		24		24		24 24	24 24		24	48	24		24	24
0.9% NSS		24														8						24							24
oxacillin		24			24			24		4			24									24							24
oxytocin																						24							
penicillin G potassium		24						24					24							24									24
phytonadione																													24
piperacillin			24			24										4						24 24							24
polymyxin B sulfate			24											24															24
potassium chloride						24							24														24		
procainamide			24											48															24
sodium bicarbonate	24		24 48	24	24										24												24 24 24	24	
tetracycline			24																										24
thiamine																													24
ticarcillin		48														24												24	
tobramycin			24														48											24	
vancomycin	24		24 48	24	24	24								24 24	24 24	24		24		24			24		24 24 24	24			24
verapamil		24																											24
vitamin B complex with C																													

MEASURING CENTRAL VENOUS PRESSURE

Your patient's central venous (CV) catheter can be used to measure his central venous pressure (CVP)—a valuable indicator of fluid status in the absence of cardiorespiratory disease. When the tricuspid valve opens, the pressure in the right atrium and the superior vena cava reflects ventricular filling pressures. Decreased pressure indicates that the patient needs fluid or has deteriorated right ventricle functioning. Conversely, elevated pressure may mean that the patient is suffering from fluid overload, or congestion and backflow pressure from left ventricular failure.

While one CVP reading may not be a true reflection of the patient's cardiac status, any trend you spot in readings taken over time may indicate an important change in the patient's condition. To ensure accuracy, three factors must remain the same for all readings: The zero point of the manometer must be level with the same spot on the patient's body; the patient must be in the same phase of his respiratory cycle; and the patient must be in the same position.

Measurements taken with the patient supine may be the most accurate, but not all patients can tolerate this position. If you elevate the patient's head, make sure you do this for

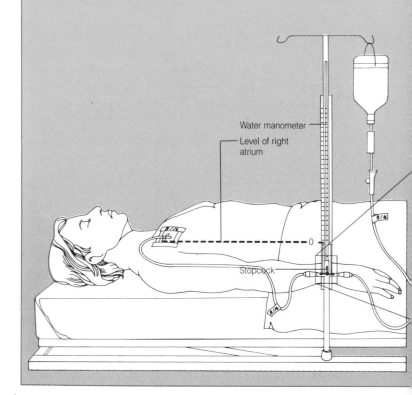

Water manometer

Level of right atrium

0

Stopcock

all readings; intrathoracic pressures can change dramatically with the patient's position.

To measure CVP, follow these guidelines:

• After you position the patient, connect the distal end of the I.V. tubing to a water manometer. If necessary, add an extension set and clear the tubing of air.

• Next, locate the level of the right atrium. Mark this area with an indelible marker so all readings are taken at this level. The zero point of the manometer should be level with the right atrium.

• Fill the water manometer to about 30 cm (or 10 cm higher than the previ-

ously recorded reading) by turning the stopcock off toward the patient and open to the manometer (1). Recheck the zero point on the manometer; it should be level with the right atrium.

• Turn the stopcock off to the I.V. fluid, so that it's now open to the patient and the manometer (2). You should see the column of water dropping with gentle fluctuations, reflecting the normal changes in intrathoracic pressure from breathing. When the water settles, record this level as the CVP.

• After you've obtained the recording, turn the stopcock off to the manometer and open to the I.V. fluid and the patient, to resume the infusion (3).

STOPCOCK POSITIONS

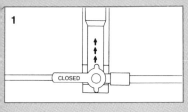

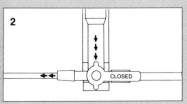

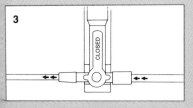

ESTIMATING BODY SURFACE AREA IN CHILDREN

Pediatric drug dosages should be calculated on the basis of body surface area or body weight. If a child is of average size, find his weight and corresponding surface area on the scale to the left. Otherwise, use the nomogram to the right: Lay a straightedge on the height and weight points for your patient, and note where it intersects on the surface area scale at center.

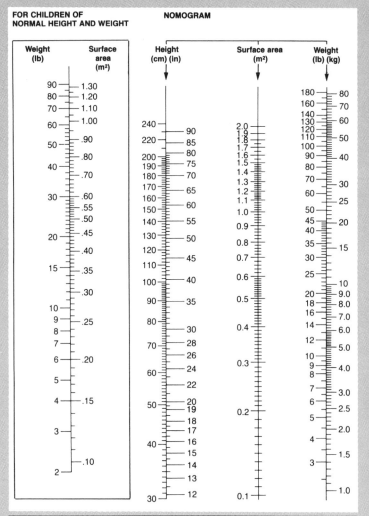

FOR CHILDREN OF NORMAL HEIGHT AND WEIGHT

NOMOGRAM

Reproduced from *Nelson Textbook of Pediatrics*, 13th edition. Courtesy W.B. Saunders Co., Philadelphia, Pa.

INDEX

i refers to an illustration; t refers to a table.